DR. WILLIAM A. CHEATHAM

TENNESSEE'S FIRST MENTAL HEALTH PROFESSIONAL

by Kay Baker Gaston

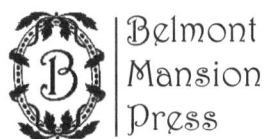

On the Front Cover –
William A. Cheatham.
Courtesy of Mary Parrent Taylor.

Tennessee Insane Asylum.
Courtesy of the Tennessee State
Library and Archives.

On the Back Cover –
Left - William A. Cheatham.
Courtesy of Bettie Thomas Chester
and Susan Chester Snow.

Right – Cheatham's second wife, Adelicia.
From the collection of the
Belmont Mansion Association.

Copyright – 2021
First Edition

Published by the
Belmont Mansion Association
Nashville, Tennessee

This book has been edited and updated by the author and was originally presented as a thesis to the Graduate Faculty of Middle Tennessee State University in partial fulfillment of the requirements for the degree Master of Arts in August 1989.

Layout and design by Danielle M. Ullrich

TABLE OF CONTENTS

ACKNOWLEDGEMENTS v

1. INTRODUCTION 1

2. ORIGINS AND EARLY YEARS 5

3. DR. CHEATHAM AS SUPERINTENDENT OF THE TENNESSEE HOSPITAL FOR THE INSANE 13

4. AN EVALUATION OF DR. CHEATHAM AND THE TENNESSEE HOSPITAL FOR THE INSANE, 1852-1862 37

5. DISRUPTION: THE IMPACT OF THE UNION OCCUPATION ON THE LIFE AND CAREER OF DR. CHEATHAM 49

6. WHEN THE WAR WAS OVER: DR. CHEATHAM AND ADELICIA ACKLEN DURING RECONSTRUCTION AND THE GILDED AGE 79

BIBLIOGRAPHY 97

ACKNOWLEDGEMENTS

I wish especially to thank my friend and thesis advisor, Dr. Robert L. Taylor, for his help in the selection and development of this topic. I am also grateful to James Henry Taylor, Robertson County historian, whose private collection of Robertson County papers and books stimulated my interest in the Cheatham family.

My Signal Mountain neighbor, Bettie Thomas Chester, gave me access to Cheatham-Ready family information along with a great deal of encouragement. Fellow descendants Martha Williamson Bradley and Mary Williamson Parrent shared their collection of letters and family stories. I also appreciate the assistance of Ridley and Irene Jackson Wills and of Elizabeth Craig Weaver Proctor. Finally, I wish to thank Mr. and Mrs. Andrew C. Buddenhagen of Murfreesboro for allowing me to review their collection of Ready papers.

Mark Brown gave me access to the papers at Belmont Mansion. I appreciate also the use of papers from the John Hunt Morgan collections of the Southern Historical Society, University of North Carolina at Chapel Hill, and the Western Kentucky University manuscript division at Bowling Green, Kentucky. I am grateful for the permission of the Houghton Library at Harvard University to cite five letters from the Dorothea L. Dix collection, as well as the help of Michael P. Musick in the Military Reference Branch of the National Archives, Washington, D. C.

Other faculty members, in addition to Dr. Taylor, who have given me assistance on this project are Dr. Sarah Howell, Dr. David L. Rowe, and Dr. Norman B. Ferris.

CHAPTER 1
INTRODUCTION

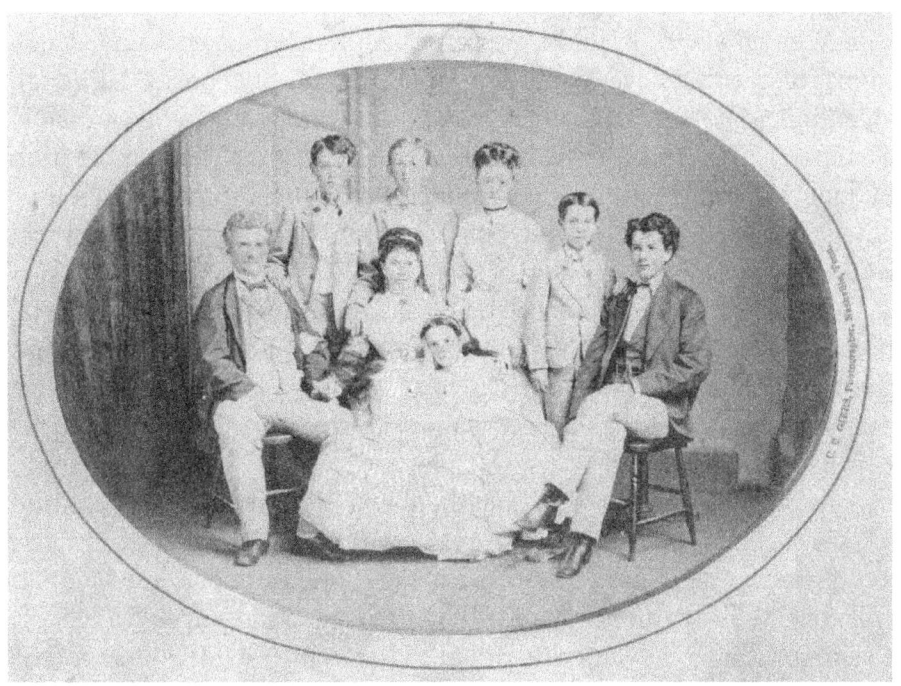

Dr. William Cheatham, Adelicia Acklen, and their blended family. C. 1867 by C. C. Giers. Courtesy of a private collection.

A mong the Washington Family Papers in the Tennessee State Library & Archives is this unsigned, handwritten note to George Augustine Washington II, who was researching the history of the Cheatham branch of his family:

> Dear George[,] Here is a picture of Cousin Billy Cheatham. He was[,] as you know[,] Cousin Mattie Weaver's father. I remember the old man very well. He lived with them on the Murfreesboro Pike after the widow Acklen at Belmont sent him home. He was her third husband.[1]

---

[1] Washington Family Papers, Tennessee State Library & Archives, Nashville: XVII-J-6, Box 140, F. 6.

If a member of his own family dismissed Dr. William Archer Cheatham in this disparaging way, perhaps it is no wonder that history has relegated him to obscurity. The widow Acklen who "sent him home" was Adelicia Hayes Franklin Acklen Cheatham who, according to one interpreter, could have "eaten Scarlet O'Hara for breakfast."[2] Although so militant a portrait of Adelicia may be unfair, she was unquestionably a woman of immense spunk, intelligence, and wealth. This combination of qualities would certainly have made her a match for the redoubtable, albeit fictitious, Scarlet, and possibly more than one for her third husband.

Nonetheless, a posterity which allows the dazzling Adelicia, notable for her style, beauty, and love of society and travel, to eclipse the more solid accomplishments of her third husband does itself a disservice. It is one that I shall attempt to rectify, although not at the expense of Adelicia.

My reappraisal of Dr. Cheatham will begin with an examination of his origins among the landed gentry of Robertson County, Tennessee, and his early career as a general practitioner of medicine. It will continue with an account of the ten-year period during which Dr. Cheatham served as Superintendent of the Tennessee Hospital for the Insane. The reappraisal will then evaluate Dr. Cheatham and the Tennessee Hospital for the Insane during the period 1852-1862 in contexts of the reform movement, the program of moral treatment which was offered there, and professional recognition. It will then turn to the disruptive impact of the Civil War and the Union occupation of Middle Tennessee on Dr. Cheatham's private life and public career. Returning to his relationship with Adelicia, in which Dr. Cheatham was a more active partner than has been previously supposed, it will conclude with a summing up of his contribution as Tennessee's first mental health professional to achieve regional and national stature.

Dr. Cheatham's career represents the flowering of a culture that was abruptly cut off in full bloom by a war, the product of both outside and inside circumstances, bringing defeat and devastation. The culture

---

[2] Roger J. Kennedy, <u>Architecture, Men, Women and Money in America, 1600-1860</u> (New York: Random House, 1985), 314.

sent off new shoots, but none duplicated the luxuriant old growth. The passage of time and the unfolding of two or three new generations could restore a measure of prosperity, but the old culture was gone forever.

    Nashvillians continued to respect the old gentleman for his education, refined manners, and professional dedication.   They remembered his association with the spectacular entertainments and immense wealth of the widow who became his second wife. But they lost any understanding or remembrance of his true significance. He became like one of the ancient trees left standing on the grounds of the state mental institution on Murfreesboro Road, long after the building which housed his innovative programs was blown to the ground. Few remembered that Dr. Cheatham planted those trees, just as he and other dedicated reformers and physicians planted the seeds of today's advancements in the treatment of mental illness. That contribution makes his a life worth reappraising.

Dr. William Cheatham. C. 1860. Courtesy of Mary Parrent Taylor.

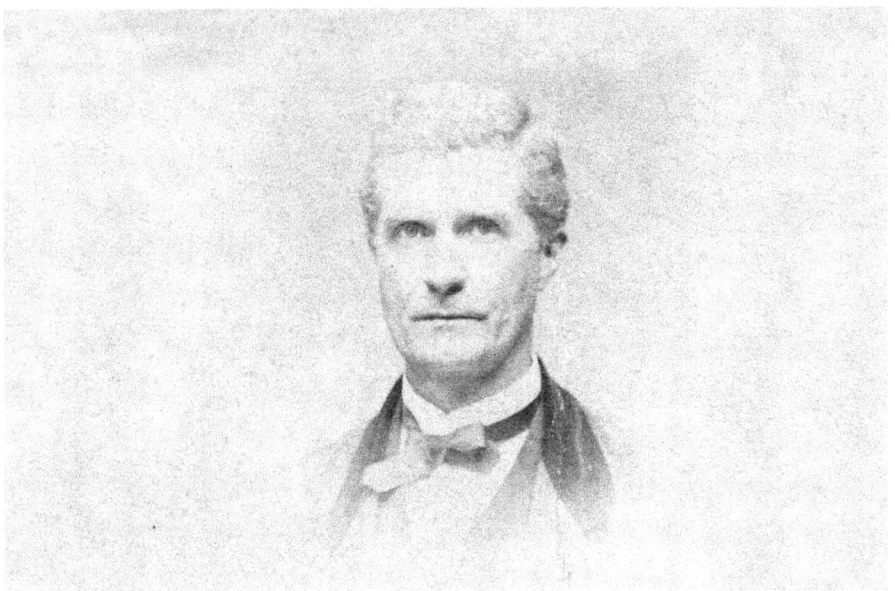

CHAPTER 2
ORIGINS AND EARLY YEARS

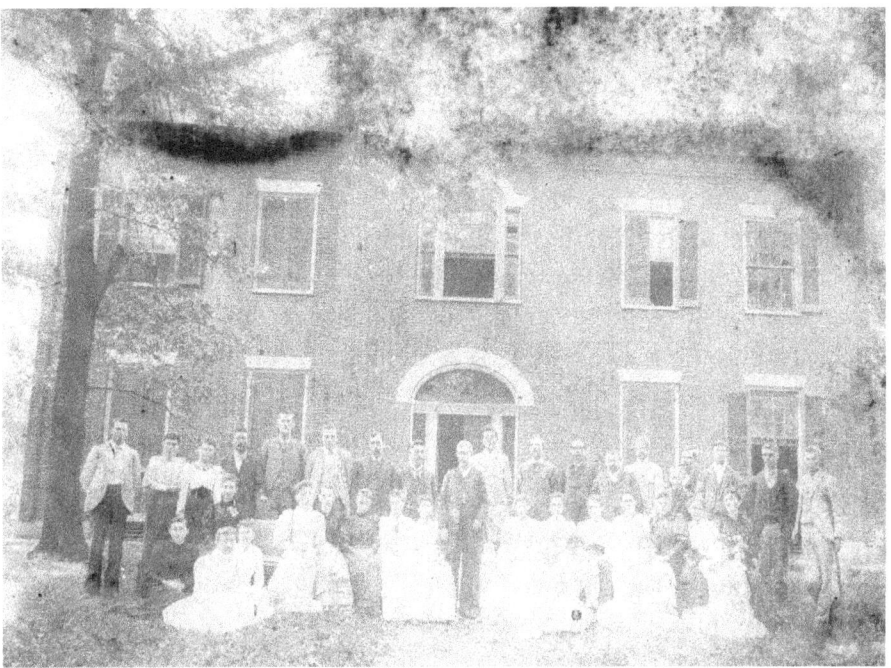

"Mansfield" the Cheatham family home constructed in 1833. Courtesy of the Robertson County Archives.

William Archer Cheatham was born into the kind of family that would have expected him to succeed. " Open a vein of almost any individual member of an old Nashville family and at least one drop of Cheatham blood will flow, so intermingled by marriage are the Cheathams with the best people of the place," wrote Octavia Zollicoffer Bond in 1909.[1] This does not appear to have been an exaggeration.

Archer Cheatham, Sr., great-grandfather of William A. Cheatham, arrived in what was then Tennessee County, North Carolina, from Amelia County, Virginia, about 1788.[2] After the establishment of

---

[1] Octavia Zollicoffer Bond, "Yester Nashville Names: The Cheatham Family," Nashville American, 22 August 1909.
[2] George Augustine Washington II, Genealogical Chart, Washington Family Papers, Tennessee State Library & Archives, Nashville, XVII-J-6, Box 140, F. 6:

Robertson County and passage of an act naming the county seat Springfield on April 20, 1796, he sold thirty acres for one hundred cents to comprise the western half of the town which would become the seat of Robertson County, Tennessee. Both Archer Cheatham and his son, Archer, Jr., were among the first purchasers of town lots for $8 apiece in 1799; in 1804 the family of Archer, Jr., was one of only four families yet residing in Springfield.[3]

Suzannah Long, the first wife of Archer, Jr., added to the Cheatham genealogy a strain of prized Washington ancestry. She was the daughter of John Long of Northampton County, North Carolina, and his wife Joyce Washington, great-great-granddaughter of Lawrence Washington and Margaret Butler, the English great-great-great-grandparents of George Washington, President of the United States.[4]

Among the children of Archer, Jr., and Suzannah Long Cheatham was Richard Cheatham, a general in the state militia who fathered eleven children. His wife, who outlived him by almost twenty years, was Susan Saunders (1801-1864), daughter of Edward Saunders of North Carolina and Elizabeth

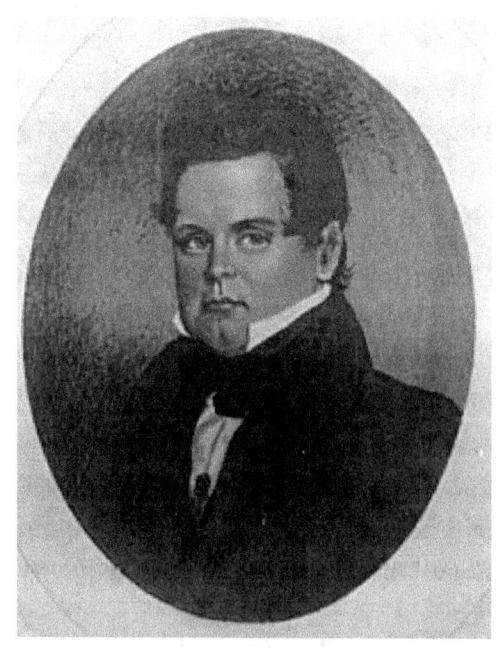

General Richard Cheatham – Father of William Archer Cheatham. Courtesy of a private collection.

---

[3] <u>Goodspeed Histories of Montgomery, Robertson, Humphreys, Stewart, Dickson, Cheatham, Houston Counties of Tennessee</u> (Columbia, Tenn., 1975), 835, 840; Charles H. Love, <u>Springfield s First 100 Years</u>, Robertson County Times, 1-2.
[4] "Data of Washington Ancestry," chart in the possession of Irene Jackson Wills, Nashville; Washington Genealogical Chart; Bettie Thomas Chester of Signal Mountain, Tennessee, interview by author, March 1988.

Williams. The second child and second son of Richard and Susan Saunders Cheatham was William Archer Cheatham, born in Springfield on August 6, 1820.[5]

General Richard Cheatham had a mercantile business, a cotton gin and gristmill, and farming and livestock interests in Robertson County, as well as a half-interest in the Sycamore Powder Mills in what later became Cheatham County. He represented Robertson County in the state legislature between 1825-1833 and 1843-45, as well as in the Constitutional Convention of 1834. In 1837 he won election as a Whig to the U. S. House of Representatives, serving one term.[6] During this time, his family and that of Senator Ephraim H. Foster resided together in Washington, D.C., along with the family of John Bell of Tennessee, then serving as Speaker of the U. S. House of Representatives.[7]

In 1833 General Cheatham constructed a fine brick house on one of the town lots his father had purchased in Springfield. Called "Mansfield," it remained in the Cheatham family until 1878.[8] In 1843 he became a trustee of Liberty Academy,[9] which his sons and possibly his daughters attended.

In sum, General Richard Cheatham was a successful, energetic man who built a substantial estate and a fine reputation, both as a businessman and a public servant. His sons were born and educated to lead, and his daughters were raised to marry well. They fulfilled his expectations to a remarkable degree.

The eldest son, Edward Saunders Cheatham (1818-1878), most closely followed in his father's footsteps, making his home in Springfield and engaging in diverse business interests as well as in politics. He represented Robertson County in the Tennessee House of Representatives, 1853-55, and served in the Senate during the 31st and

---

[5] Washington Genealogical Chart. Elizabeth Williams Saunders was half-sister to the third wife of her father-in-law, Archer Cheatham, Jr.

[6] Biographical Directory, Tennessee General Assembly 1796-1967, Robertson County (Preliminary),Tennessee State Library & Archives, 7-8.

[7] "R. Cheatham Genealogy," Washington Family Papers, XVII-J-6, Box 140, F. 6. The source of this information is Verner M. Jones in a letter to Kitty Cheatham dated 31 December 1932.

[8] Deborah Kelley Henderson, Robertson County's Heritage of Homes (Springfield: Robertson County Antiquities Foundation, 1979), 38-39.

[9] Biographical Directory, 8.

34th General Assemblies, 1855-57 and 1861-63 (Confederate). He was Speaker of the Senate in both sessions. Cheatham County, established during the 31st General Assembly, was named in his honor. Early in 1862, after the fall of Fort Donelson, it fell to him as Speaker of the Senate to gather up the State papers and other valuable documents and convey them South.[10]

Edward S. Cheatham was also the organizer and president of the Edgefield & Kentucky Railroad, which ran from Edgefield, a suburb of Nashville, by way of Springfield to the Kentucky line at Guthrie, in 1860-61. Like his father, he served as trustee of Liberty Academy, which he attended prior to the University of Nashville. Like most members of his family, he married well. His first wife was Jane Ellen Foster, daughter of family friend Ephraim H. Foster; his second was Julia Cockrill, daughter of famed agriculturalist Mark R. Cockrill; and his third was Lottie Wall of Holly Springs, Mississippi.[11]

William Archer Cheatham, as second son, was perhaps freer than his older brother to pursue studious inclinations. After attending Liberty Academy, he studied medicine at the University of Nashville and then at the University of Pennsylvania, graduating in March of 1843. He was unquestionably among the best educated doctors in the state when he returned to Springfield to open his practice.

One of his first cases was a referral from George Augustine Washington of "Wessyngton,"his relative both by descent and by the marriage of his aunt, Mary Cheatham, to Joseph Washington, George Augustine's father. On June 30, 1843, the young Dr. Cheatham addressed a note to his cousin, who was five years his senior, prescribing a preparation of acetate of lead dissolved in rose water to treat a nursing mother whose breast had become infected.[12]

A year and a half later, on January 1, 1845, Dr. Cheatham moved to Nashville. There he earned the regard of his fellow physicians, as evidenced by his appointment as a delegate of the Medical Society of Tennessee at the great medical convention to be held in New York City

---

[10] Ibid., 6-7; A. L. Dorsey, "Historical Events of Past Hundred Years," from the collection of James Henry Taylor, Springfield, Tennessee; Bond, 2.

[11] Biographical Directory, 6; Washington Genealogical Chart.

[12] Dr. William A. Cheatham to George Augustine Washington, 30 June 1843, Washington Family Papers, XVII-F-6, Box 32, F. 61.

on May 5, 1846. Accompanying him was his sister, Martha Washington Cheatham (b. 1827), "having concluded that the trip would be more pleasant and profitable to her than one to New Orleans," where she would otherwise have accompanied their brother Edward.

Dr. Cheatham made this report in a letter to his cousin, George Augustine Washington, dating it April 17, 1846, from the steamboat "Magic" near Louisville, Kentucky. It was an unexpected trip, and he had questioned the propriety of leaving home. But, after being urged by many of his friends, he became convinced that it would be of advantage to him professionally, and he had therefore embarked with apparent satisfaction.[13]

The concluding paragraph of the letter to his cousin George had contained a bit of Nashville gossip about various couples planning to marry. Before long he would be among those young married couples who interested him so strongly. On October 20, 1846, William Archer Cheatham married Mary Emma Ready of Murfreesboro.[14]

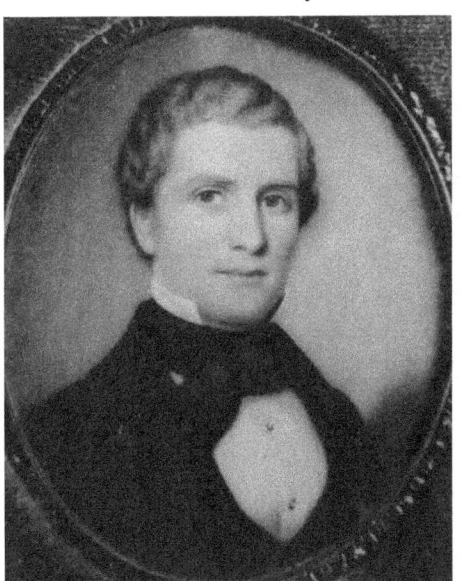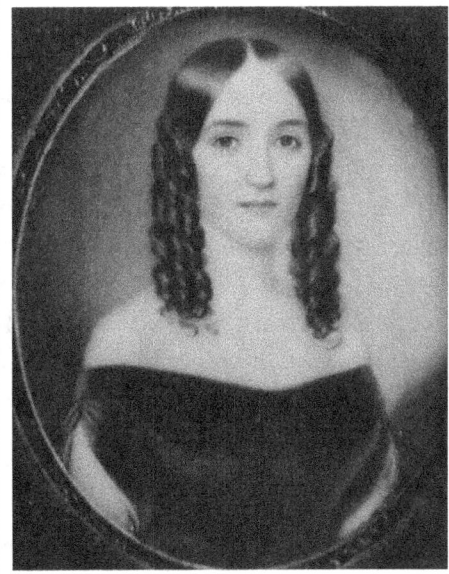

Left: William Archer Cheatham (1820-1900), c. 1846.
Right: Mary Emma Ready Cheatham (1827-1864), c. 1846.
Both images courtesy of a private collection.

---

[13] Dr. William A. Cheatham to George Augustine Washington, 17 April 1846, Washington Family Papers, XVII-F-6, Box 32, F. 61.
[14] Washington Genealogical Chart.

Born on August 23, 1827, Mary Ready was only nineteen, seven years her husband's junior. She was one of five children—four daughters and a son--of Charles Ready, a prominent lawyer and planter, and his wife, Martha Strong. In the 1890s Miss Jane Thomas recalled how, in 1822, Miss Lavinia King and Miss Martha Strong had come to Nashville to spend the winter. "The legislature was in session, and a young lawyer named Ready, from Murfreesboro, was a legislator," she wrote. "He fell in love with and married Miss Mattie Strong."[15]

The Readys lived in a large, two-story brick house on East Main Street, near the public square in Murfreesboro. Like Richard Cheatham, Charles Ready was a Whig, and active in politics; from 1853 to 1859 he would serve as a United States congressman.[16] Like the Cheathams in Robertson County, the Readys were a "first family" of Rutherford County. Mary Cheatham's grandfather, Colonel Charles Ready, had built "The Corners," one of the first brick houses in the county, on his plantation near Readyville in 1804.[17]

Miss Jane Thomas remembered Mary Ready Cheatham as a "beautiful, refined, elegant woman." She recalled that when the Cheathams were first married "they lived on the north corner of Summer and Cedar Streets, in a two-story brick house built by George Yearger."[18] They eventually had two children. Martha Strong Cheatham was born on January 24, 1853, and Richard M. Cheatham was born on July 8, 1855.[19] Like both their families, William and Mary Cheatham were Presbyterians and Whigs. They almost certainly took an active part in the political, intellectual, and social life of antebellum Nashville.

Professionally, Dr. Cheatham associated in practice first with Dr. Thomas Buchanan and later with Dr. W. K. Bowling,[20] both

---

[15] Miss Jane H. Thomas, Old Days in Nashville, Tenn. Reminiscences. Reprinted from the Nashville Daily American, 1895-96 (Nashville, Tenn.: Publishing House Methodist Episcopal Church, South, 1897), 54.
[16] James A. Ramage, Rebel Raider: The Life of General John Hunt Morgan (Lexington: The University Press of Kentucky, 1986), 57.
[17] Mary B. Hughes, Hearthstones: The Story of Historic Rutherford County Homes (Murfreesboro: Mid-South Publishing Co., 1942), 16.
[18] Thomas, 54.
[19] "Data of Washington Ancestry," Irene Jackson Wills.
[20] Nashville American, 11 June 1900, 8.

prominent in Nashville medical and social circles. Dr. Bowling was William A. Cheatham's step-uncle, having married Melissa Saunders Cheatham, the widow of his uncle, John Long Cheatham, after his untimely death on October 12, 1833.[21] Dr. Bowling was step-father to the four children of John Long Cheatham, one of whom, his father's namesake, became a physician and entered practice with Dr. Bowling in 1855. The Bowlings also had a daughter of their own, Powhattan Bowling.[22] Thus William A. Cheatham's practice of medicine with Dr. Bowling was virtually a family affair.

Dr. Bowling, in addition to maintaining a private practice, was also a professor in the University of Nashville Medical Department and served on the board of the state hospital for the insane. He may have been influential both in securing and in persuading Dr. Cheatham to accept an eight-year appointment as Physician and Superintendent of the new Tennessee Hospital for the Insane, beginning in 1852.

---

[21] Washington Genealogical Chart.
[22] Obsequies of John L. Cheatham, M.D. of Nashville, Tennessee, with an address by J.B. Ferguson (Nashville: John T. S. Fall, 1863); Washington Genealogical Chart.

CHAPTER 3
DR. CHEATHAM AS SUPERINTENDENT OF THE TENNESSEE HOSPITAL FOR THE INSANE

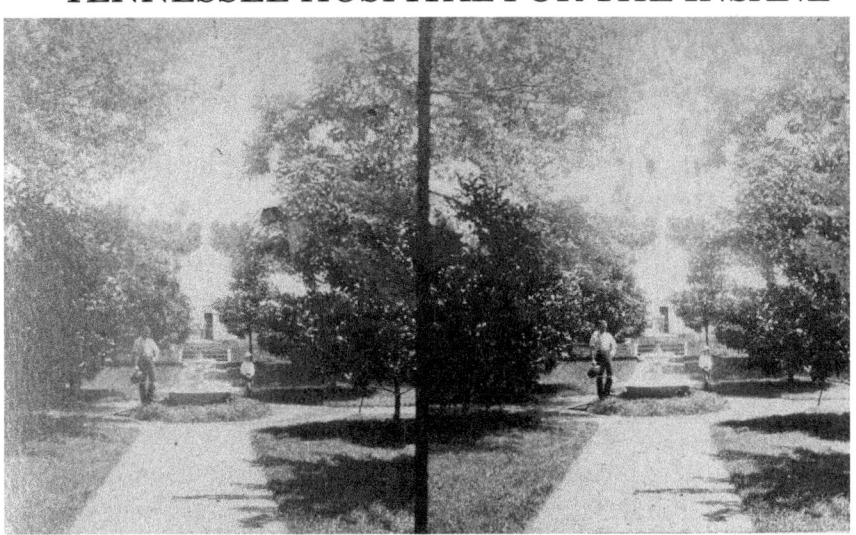

Stereoview image of the Tennessee Insane Asylum grounds, by C. C. Giers. C. 1884. Courtesy of the Tennessee State Library and Archives.

Throughout the United States, the period 1825 to 1865 witnessed tremendous growth in publicly owned asylums, mostly state-supported, from nine to thirty-two. Although mental illness was a recognized specialty by the 1840s, the terms "psychiatry" and "psychiatrist" were not in general use until the twentieth century. If we use the word "psychiatrist," we are referring to physicians who served mental hospitals as superintendents, assistant superintendents, or visiting physicians. They had a virtual monopoly on the care of the mentally ill. "At most, their number never exceeded two hundred, and for much of the time before 1865 it fell short of half that sum," writes Norman Dain in <u>Concepts of Insanity</u>. "The leaders of the profession, the asylum superintendents, constituted a small, select group whose medical education and public and professional standing were superior to other medical practitioners."[1]

Although the superintendents compiled statistics, they rarely conducted scientific research as we know it today, and were not noted as a group for their intellectual achievements; their reputation grew out of "their ability as organizers and administrators of hospitals that practiced the latest techniques of treatment."[2] These physicians were ruled by a spirit of optimism; "yet despite their faith in mankind, psychiatrists generally were not naive or impractical; they were worldly, capable, and intelligent."[3]

Some historians are more impressed with their accomplishments than others. Albert Deutsch, in <u>The Mentally Ill in America; A History of Their Care and Treatment From Colonial Times</u>, writes:

> It is significant that the greatest reforms in the care and treatment of the insane in the first half of the nineteenth century lay rather in the substitution of kind for cruel treatment than in scientific therapy. Even the most advanced hospitals of the day resembled well-conducted boarding houses rather than hospitals.[4]

But Norman Dain gives early asylums credit for a therapeutic approach similar to today's milieu therapy.[5]

In any evaluation of what came to be called psychiatry during the first half of the nineteenth century, it is important to understand that

---

[1] Norman Dain, <u>Concepts of Insanity in the United States, 1789- 1865</u> (New Brunswick, NJ: Rutgers University Press, 1964), 55.
[2] Ibid., 56.
[3] Ibid., 59.
[4] Albert Deutsch, <u>The Mentally Ill in America: A History of Their Care and Treatment from Colonial Times</u>, 2d ed. (New York: Columbia University Press, 1949), 188.
[5] Dain, 115. Development of milieu or social therapy for mental patients occurred after World War II. It grew out of the recognition that all aspects of the clinical environment had therapeutic possibilities, particularly group interaction.

the intellectual leaders in this pioneer generation of American psychiatry--men like Issac Ray, Thomas Kirkbride, Samuel Woodward, and Amariah Brigham--had no formal training in psychiatry; there was, of course, none to be had. They were, however, humanitarians and, necessarily, optimists, deeply concerned with ameliorating the lot of the mentally ill and encouraging the hope that insanity might be curable. Not surprisingly, they were receptive to any theoretical innovation that implied a more hopeful view of the nature of mental illness and the possibility of cure.[6]

Constance M. McGovern, in Masters of Madness: Social Origins of the American Psychiatric Association, points out that "none of the doctors who headed the new asylums and implemented the new therapy had set out to devote their lives to the insane."[7] William A. Cheatham was among this number. Fortunately, he had received the best medical education possible in his day, having graduated from the University Of Pennsylvania School Of Medicine in Philadelphia in March, 1843. This was "a mecca of medical education in the first half of the nineteenth century," the only medical school besides the College of Physicians and Surgeons in New York City offering adequate clinical experience to students.[8]

In 1860, William A. Cheatham was one of only 83 doctors who had chosen new careers as superintendents of American hospitals for the insane as "changing attitudes about the insane, the emerging medical model, and the optimism about the plan of moral treatment converged with the needs and aspirations of at least these eighty-three men, making them receptive to the new field."[9] Asylum administration was a professional risk because of lack of preparation and training, yet it also held an appeal for those with humanitarian instincts and a penchant for living on the edge. "I am over head and ears in business,

---

[6] Charles E. Rosenberg, The Trial of the Assassin Guiteau: Psychiatry and Law in the Gilded Age (Chicago: University of Chicago Press, 1968), 61.
[7] Constance M. McGovern, Masters of Madness: Social Origins of the American Psychiatric Profession (Hanover, NH: University Press of New England, 1985), 43.
[8] Ibid., 47-48.
[9] Ibid., 56.

one would think the world was going crazy. By the by this thing of piloting a lunatic asylum requires steady nerves," wrote Dr. William M. Awl to Dr. Samuel B. Woodward on April 18, 1842.[10]

One year after Awl's letter to Woodward, William A. Cheatham graduated from the University of Pennsylvania Medical School and established his practice, first in his birthplace of Springfield in Robertson County, Tennessee, and, within the next year, in Nashville. In May of 1845 he attended the 16th Annual Meeting of the Medical Society of Tennessee. The following year he was excused because he was attending the National Medical Convention in New York as a delegate of the Tennessee Society. In May, 1847, Cheatham, with Dr J. W. Percy, was appointed secretary of the Medical Convention of the State of Tennessee. By 1850, however, he was no longer regularly attending meetings of the State Medical Society.[11] His new professional affiliation would be with the Association of Medical Superintendents of American Institutions for the Insane, the AMSAII. Founded in 1844, it was "the only established organization of medical experts in psychiatric matters."[12]

In March of 1852, when Dr. William A. Cheatham officially left the private practice of medicine to assume his new post as Superintendent of the Tennessee Hospital for the Insane, he was well versed in every aspect of his profession but had no particular qualifications for treating the mentally ill beyond those acquired by

---

[10] Ibid., 62. Dr. Awl was Superintendent of the Ohio Lunatic Asylum and Dr. Woodward was Superintendent of the Worchester State Hospital in Worcester, Massachusetts; both were founding members of the Association of Medical Superintendents of American Institutions for the Insane, forerunner of the American Psychiatric Association, in 1844. Deutsch, 191.

[11] Proceedings of the Medical Society of the State of Tennessee at the 16th Annual Meeting (Nashville: Cameron & Fall, 1845); Proceedings, etc., at the 17th Annual Meeting (Nashville: Burton, Billings & Fall, 1846); Proceedings of the Medical Convention of the State of Tennessee (Nashville: E. R. Glascock & Co., 1847); Proceedings of the 21st Annual Meeting of the Tennessee Medical Society (Murfreesborough, April, 1850); Transactions of the Tennessee State Medical Society (Nashville: J. F. Morgan, 1853); Transactions of the 27th Annual Session of the Tennessee Medical Society (Nashville: Cameron & Fall, 1856); Transactions of the 29th Annual Meeting of the Tennessee Medical Society (Nashville: T. S. Fall, 1858).

[12] Rosenberg, 61.

most physicians of his day. From that time forward, however, he "devoted most of his time to the study of insanity and treatment of the insane," his success winning for him "distinction and renown throughout the state."[13] In this context he would qualify as Tennessee's first mental health professional.

Clearly the trustees had Dr. Cheatham in mind when they requested, in their report to the legislature of October, 1851, two amendments to the Act of 1848 authorizing construction of the new hospital on Murfreesboro Pike. First, they asked the legislature to remove the stipulation that the superintendent reside with his family in the hospital and that his wife perform the duties of matron. "This limitation on the powers of the Board of Trustees will, we fear, be found very injudicious, and greatly contract the number of those persons from whom a proper selection of superintendent can be made," board chairman Alex Allison stated in his 1851 report to the General Assembly. "The office is one requiring extraordinary qualifications, and the combination of rare qualities which will be necessary . . . can be found in but few individuals."[14] The board requested permission, which was granted, to hire a matron who would be willing to reside in the institution, enabling the physician and his family to occupy a building situated a small distance from the asylum, yet convenient to it.

A second request, not immediately granted, was for the salary of a gardener or horticulturist to supervise and manage the farm on which the new institution was located. The rationale for this request closely reflects the philosophy of Dr. Cheatham, who was deeply interested in horticulture, particularly as it related to mental health. The basic concept was that the institution would raise its own food on the farm, with the help of patients who were willing and able to work. At the same time "the improvement and beautification of the premises" would be a therapeutic factor in relieving depression among the patients "and assist greatly in recalling and strengthening their shattered intellects."[15]

---

[13] Nashville American, 11 June 1900, 8.
[14] Report of the Commissioners, in Relation to the State Hospital for the Insane in Tennessee, to the General Assembly of the State of Tennessee (Nashville: w. F. Bang & Co., Printers, 1851), 5.
[15] Ibid., 6.

By December of 1851 Dr. Cheatham was actively laying the groundwork to assume his post, as evidenced by the following letter to reformer Dorothea L. Dix, who had instigated the project with her memorial to the legislature in 1847:

Philad[elphi]a Dec. 18th[,] 1851

My dear Miss Dix,

Since I saw you I have passed three days pleasantly and, I trust profitably, with Dr. Kirkbride. It was my intention to leave here this morning for Harrisburg, but the precarious state of Mrs. Cheatham's health prevented me. The intensely cold weather forced me to seek a more genial climate as soon as possible. Tomorrow morning, if Mrs. C. is well enough, I shall leave here, via Charleston, for home. Miss Sharpless had been engaged as Supervisor of the female wards, by Dr. Kirkbride. The Dr. promised to use his influence in inducing her to visit Tennessee. I hope, with your assistance, there will be no difficulty in accomplishing it. Dr. K. could think of no man, whom he could recommend as supervisor of the male wards. Will you think of this & if anyone is suggested to your mind inform me of it as soon as possible. I would be glad if you could visit Tennessee before the adjournment of the present Legislature. Many things ought to be done before patients can be properly classified or even made as comfortable as they should be in the new institution. If you could be there, I am satisfied, the present Legislature would not hesitate to do anything you would ask of them. Think of this, my dear Miss Dix, & do come, if possible, sometime during the month of January. If you cannot come at that time do come as soon as you can. It is so very important to commence right. I will write as soon as I reach home. Please write & let me know where to direct my letters.

Yours very truly,
W. A. Cheatham[16]

---

[16] William A. Cheatham to Dorothea L. Dix, 18 December 1851, Houghton Library of Harvard University, b ms Am 1838 (135). Dr. Thomas A. Kirkbride was

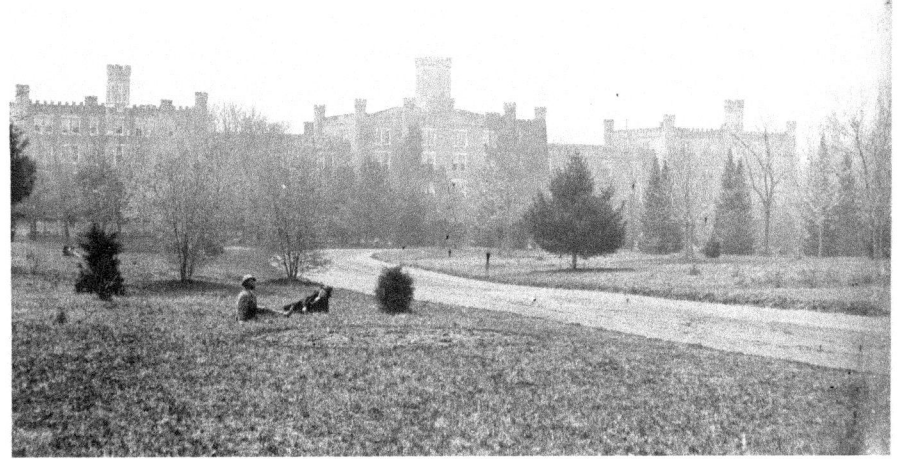

Tennessee Insane Asylum, by Calvert. Courtesy of the Tennessee State Library and Archives.

Meanwhile the new building, designed by architect Adolphus Heiman, was nearing completion. Dr. Cheatham defined the style of architecture as "castellated," an appropriate designation for a structure boasting fourteen octagonal towers.[17] As described by a Mr. Allison, the hospital consisted of a four-story central section measuring 95 by 50 feet, and two lines of wards, each three stories high and 76 feet long, with two four-story end buildings measuring 36 by 56. Connected together, they formed a line of walls 325 feet long. The structure housed 138 apartments, or rooms, including single and double wards, dormitories, dining rooms, water closets, and areas for various domestic purposes, connected by about 800 feet of passages.[18]

Allison described a heating system utilizing basement furnaces with conductors and flues to carry heat throughout the building and ventilate it. A small steam engine was designed to pump water from a

---

Superintendent of the Pennsylvania Hospital for the Insane. He had the greatest success with moral treatment, probably because he limited the entrance and retention of chronic patients, and also because his institution was financially independent. David J. Rothman, The Discovery of the Asylum: Social Order and Disorder in the New Republic (Boston: Little, Brown and Company, 1971), 280.

[17] Reports of the Trustees, Treasurer and Physician of the Tennessee Hospital for the Insane, Transmitted to the Legislature on the Sixth November, 1853 (Nashville: Union and American Steam Press, 1853), 10-11.

[18] Report of the Commissioners (1851), 4.

reservoir through iron pipes to a tank on top of the building, where it could be distributed to various locations. Sewers, or drains, were cut from each end of the building to carry off water and filth. Tin covered the superstructure and cast iron sashes secured the windows. The $75,000 which the legislature had appropriated to build the hospital was not sufficient to construct 20 or 30 lodges for noisy patients apart from the main building, so the basement rooms were converted to this purpose for the time being.[19]

On February 24, 1853, Dr. Cheatham again reported to Miss Dix:

> On 1st March last I entered upon my official duties. The patients, 60 in number, were at that time in the old building in the vicinity of Nashville. I was compelled to commence with every position filled by inexperienced persons; not one had ever been connected with an institution before. The miserable condition of the patients, couple with the inexperience of all presented difficulties which cannot be imagined[,] much less described. Finding that I could accomplish nothing in the old building I determined to occupy the new as soon as possible. Although the new was in an unfinished state any change almost was desirable.[20]

Accordingly, he removed the patients on April 19, 1852, chartering stages and an omnibus for the female patients, and transporting the male patients by rail to within one mile of the building to walk the remainder of the distance. What could have been a traumatic event "was effected without the slightest accident or difficulty, and with no noise or excitement of any kind calculated to attract attention."[21]

Despite "having gotten along astonishingly," he was concerned that the legislature, at its last session, had made no further appropriation to extend the wings of the building. They did continue a

---

[19] Ibid., 3-4.
[20] William A. Cheatham to Dorothea L. Dix, 24 February 1853, Houghton Library of Harvard University, b ms Am 1838 (135).
[21] Reports . . . of the Tennessee Hospital for the Insane (1853), 15.

tax for one year, but it had not been received into the Treasury, and thus compelling him to get by without many necessities. "We have no bath room furnished, no hot water arrangement, no servants rooms, no wash house and drying room and the water closets are nuisances, as they are now arranged," he reported to Miss Dix. "In fact innumerable things are missing to make this, what it should be, a good institution." He begged her to attend the October session of the legislature: "I know if you would come that everything necessary, to make this an institution of which the state should be proud, could be easily accomplished."[22]

There is no evidence that Miss Dix did attend the next session of the legislature. But Dr. Cheatham presented an impressive official report on the first nineteen months of operation from March 1, 1852. During that period, 176 patients were hospitalized in the new institution. He had discharged 42 of these as cured, 13 as much improved, and five as unimproved. Two had run off and nine had died, leaving 100 patients under treatment. Already the demand exceeded the capacity of the institution; 62 patients were in the male wards, which were built to accommodate 50.[23]

Cheatham was concerned that those patients able to pay for services would soon be crowded out by indigent patients, to whom the law gave preference. The state also had the power to commit the criminally insane to the institution, and five patients in this category were already there. A few patients from other states had found their way into the asylum. Finally, Cheatham mentioned "frequent applications for the admission of insane slaves," who could not be admitted because the law had made no provision for this class of patients. "A small ward for such patients, separated from the other wards, would be a humane provision," he suggested.[24]

His lengthy report included numerous tables showing the civil condition, respective ages, probable cause of insanity, number of deaths, and other factors relating to the asylum population. Although the cause of insanity in 55 out of 176 cases was unascertained, other leading categories were ill health (36), religious excitement (15),

---

[22] Cheatham to Dix, 24 February 1853.
[23] Although the asylum had been originally designed to house 250 patients, the plan had been scaled down so that its capacity was now 100 patients.
[24] Reports (1853), 18-21.

intense mental application (12), hereditary predisposition (10), and intemperance (7). Minor causes included the use of snuff, avarice, and pecuniary embarrassment.

But Cheatham was cautious in these assessments, citing Dr. Thomas Kirkbride, superintendent of the Pennsylvania Hospital for the Insane, who warned of the danger of mistaking certain habits "'for the starting point of the disease, when in reality, these habits were only some of the melancholy effects of deranged intellect.'"[25]

The new superintendent also reported on the condition of the farm, which had been allowed to deteriorate, with fences down and neighborhood thoroughfares cutting across the fields. Although April was rather late in the season to make preparations for a crop, they managed to crib 100 barrels of corn, save 2,000 bundles of oats, put up 8 tons of hay and 1,500 bundles of fodder, and raise 150 bushels of sweet potatoes, 25 bushels of Irish potatoes, and a good quantity of vegetables. The patients had done all of this work under the supervision of one attendant.

Since January 1, 1853, they had erected 2 miles of cedar picketing fence; partially graded a road from the main building to the Murfreesboro pike; planted grass and shrubbery, and laid out walks in front of the building; and dug out a cellar under the new wing presently under construction. In 1853, corn production had risen dramatically to 350 barrels, oats to 20,000 bundles, fodder to 15,000 bundles, hay to 12 tons, sweet potatoes to 500 bushels, and Irish potatoes to 250 bushels; in addition, the farm had produced 30 bushels of peas and melons, cantaloupes, and a great abundance of excellent garden vegetables. The patients raised these crops with the assistance of one attendant and two black men.

Dr. Cheatham was careful to explain that the patients worked only voluntarily, because for them work was only a type of therapy and must be classified as an amusement. Along these same lines, the female patients had made a great number of quilts, as well as clothing for themselves and the male patients. Various other amusements included reading, music, and various games; they were also encouraged to walk, go fishing, and attend church.

---

[25] Ibid., 21-30.

Cheatham graciously acknowledged several gifts of books, newspapers, and plants to the hospital, including shrubbery from his mother- in-law, Mrs. Charles Ready. He also thanked Mr. and Mrs. Cyrus Chatfield, former steward and matron at the New York State Asylum in Utica, for filling those posts so competently at the Tennessee institution.[26] Anyone reading Cheatham's report would have been impressed with its thoroughness. Without any prior experience in the field of mental illness, he had successfully transferred the patients from the old asylum to the new; statistically analyzed his patient group with a view toward achieving greater understanding of their illness and evaluating progress made; consulted a leading authority in the field, Dr. Kirkbride; turned fallow land into a productive farming operation to grow healthful food while at the same time providing fresh air and exercise for those patients who chose to work; brought in skilled professionals, Mr. and Mrs. Chatfield, to supervise the wards; and attracted private donations from prominent individuals in the community.

Cheatham concluded his first Biennial Report on October 1, 1853, by reminding the legislators that he, like others in his field, "had given the specialty of insanity only such attention as is common with the generality of practitioners," until he was "suddenly transplanted from a general and miscellaneous practice into a new field, without specific training or apprenticeship to its requirements." His success thus far had inspired him "with a determination to do whatever industry and energy --under providence-- can achieve for the amelioration of that class of unfortunate beings, which a God of mercy has submitted to his ministration."[27]

Dr. Cheatham's energy and industry would be expressed through a program of moral treatment representing the most advanced thinking of his day. According to Milton Greenblatt, in his foreword to Ruth B. Caplan's Psychiatry and the Community in Nineteenth-Century America, the most moving theme of the period

---

[26] Ibid., 31-34.
[27] Ibid., 34.

has to do with the high level of humanism, individual care, and attention accorded the mentally ill patient ... under the banner of moral treatment. The dignity of the patient was preserved and enhanced, and the conditions of his living were extraordinarily rich and culturally impressive compared with the subsequent era of custodialism that dominated for so long, and even compared with the level of care and attention that prevail today in our public mental hospitals.

He also notes that the success of moral treatment "depended on small-group living, was nourished by close inter-personal contact, and included, by its very nature, a concern with continuity of care. When this was lost, everything was lost."[28]

The philosophy of moral treatment was implemented through moral management. The basic premise was that the body could be influenced through the mind; and, further, that through education and the establishment of regular habits order could be imposed upon minds that had become alienated from society. "Moral methods" were in part a reaction against medical excesses of the past, such as restraint and blood-letting. Physicians relying on moral treatment would employ social restraints and re-education, hoping to erase or relieve the organic lesions in the brain that presumably had caused the patient to become ill in the first place.[29]

A rural location was essential to achieve the desired effect, because only in the country was there enough land for work and recreation in a healthful environment. However, patients must also be close enough to towns in order to receive visitors, obtain supplies, and receive a certain amount of cultural stimulation. The physical layout of the asylum was equally as important as the setting. Practitioners of moral treatment placed a great emphasis on a soothing atmosphere,

---

[28] Ruth B. Caplan, Psychiatry and the Community in Nineteenth Century America (New York: Basic Books, Inc., 1969), viii. In 1969, Greenblatt was serving as Commissioner of the Massachusetts Department of Mental Health; Professor of Psychiatry, Tufts School of Medicine; and Lecturer in Psychiatry, Harvard Medical School and Boston University School of Medicine.
[29] Ibid., 26, 28.

internal design, and such features as central heat, ventilation, baths, and water closets.[30]

The physician-superintendent presided over a "closely knit social system" designed to support and control the patient. Institutions functioning under the system of moral treatment were no larger than 200 beds in order to provide individual attention for all patients. The superintendent and his family usually lived in the hospital, taking meals with the patients and also taking part in recreational activities, and generally set an example of correct behavior.[31] Cheatham's family was something of an exception, in that they lived in a cottage on the grounds; but they were closely involved with the patients. Cheatham himself thought of the patients as his extended family, as indicated by his reference to many of his "household" having been attacked by illness in the summer of 1854.[32]

In October of 1855, Sterling R. Cockrill, President of the Board of Trustees, reported that construction on the two wings originally planned for the hospital was well under way. The work was being done under the direction of the architect, Major Heiman. The wing for male patients would soon be ready for occupation; but the other wing, for female patients, was just under roof. Funds for this construction had been voted at the last session of the legislature.[33]

Cockrill requested additional funds for two years in order to complete the west wing, furnish both wings, complete a new plan of steam heat and ventilation, improve the grounds, build a workshop, and open a road from the hospital to a depot on the Chattanooga and Nashville Railroad, so that a supply of coal could be brought in, and also to make the hospital more convenient to the public. He noted that, in line with the most "humane, enlightened, and eminently rational mode of treating insanity now pursued," the trustees had "expended nothing

---

[30] Ibid., 29-30.
[31] Ibid., 31.
[32] Second Biennial Reports of the Trustees, Treasurer, and the Physician and Superintendent of the Tennessee Hospital for the Insane (Nashville: B. R, McKennie & Co., 1855), 28.
[33] Ibid., 5-6.

for walls, but recommend in lieu thereof, extensive airing grounds, shrubberies, fountains, walks and sunshades."[34]

In 1855, as in 1853, Anthony Dibrell filed a Treasurer's Report; but this time he called himself "Treasurer of the Tennessee Hospital for the Insane" instead of "Treasurer of Lunatic Asylum," which may demonstrate that a new, enlightened attitude was beginning to take hold. Revenue and expenditures had more than doubled. Income of $36,433.96 had been received in 1853; in 1855 income had risen to $90,881.20; and expenditures for the periods were $33,996.74 and $90,818.20 respectively. Much of the increased expenditure was related to construction on the new wings, and the income for it came from additional appropriations from the state.[35]

Dr. Cheatham explained that the facade had been lengthened by the addition of the wings so that it now presented a front of 409 feet. The wings were three stories high exclusive of the basement, which contained a separate kitchen for each wing with dining rooms above. The violent patients would be removed from the basement of the present building and placed in rooms at the extreme end of each wing. These rooms were lined with wood and were well warmed and ventilated. Each wing contained 48 single rooms and 8 dormitories, and each was planned to accommodate 75 patients, so that the entire hospital would be able to accommodate 250 patients, as originally planned.[36]

Since the last report, when there were 100 patients in the institution, 92 additional patients had been admitted and 87 discharged or died, leaving 105 under treatment as of October 1, 1855. Of the 192 patients accommodated there in the two years since the last report, 40 had been "restored to reason and returned to their friends," and, of those, only 2 had relapsed. Cheatham believed those two had been discharged too soon. "It is frequently the case that patients after leaving the Hospital are allowed, or allow themselves, to resort to the very habits from which the disease may have originated--such as the excessive use of stimulants, &c.," Cheatham cautioned "We most earnestly advise that patients leaving the Hospital--even cured--should

---

[34] Ibid., 8-9.
[35] Reports (1853), 8-9; Second Biennial Reports (1855), 14-15.
[36] Second Biennial Reports (1855), 18-20.

refrain for a considerable time, from engaging in anything calculated to create excitement, such as religious or political meetings, &c."[37]

Cheatham again included numerous tables analyzing the patient population. He admonished the legislature for requiring that he admit insane patients from each county in the ratio of their insane population, when no county had ever made a report of its number of insane. He also noted that the law requiring him to discharge incurable cases to make room for those more responsive to treatment was wise in theory but impractical of execution. He suggested that the county authorities be required to pay the usual rates of private patients after being notified that the patient was incurable. Finally, he took advantage of this opportunity to correct an erroneous notion still held by the general population, namely, that blood-letting was an effective remedy for mania. He cited Dr. Pliny Earle, formerly superintendent and physician of the Bloomingdale Asylum in New York, in rebuttal of this practice, which had been erroneously promoted by Dr. Benjamin Rush, the first great American physician.[38]

During the last two years, the cedar picketing fences had been extended and the farm had continued to yield bumper crops. In 1854, 5,412 pounds of pork had been raised and fattened, and in 1855, 300 bushels of rye had been raised in addition to corn, oats, peas, potatoes, and almost every variety of vegetable. The patients, again supervised by their attendants and two black men in 1854, three in 1855, had done all of this work, in addition to excavating the basement of the east wing in 1854 and the west wing in 1855. Cheatham noted that pasturage had regularly supported from 10 to 12 cows, which supplied an abundance of milk.

Cheatham thanked various newspapers for sending copies free of charge, and acknowledged the gift of public documents from his father-in-law, Hon. Charles Ready, and Hon. F. K. Zollicoffer.[39] He noted that relations with the trustees had been "most agreeable and

---

[37] Ibid., 23-26.

[38] Ibid., 30-45.

[39] Felix K. Zollicoffer (1812- 1862) was elected to Congress in 1852 and served in the House of Representatives until 1859. A states- rights Whig, he was known as "Tennessee's 'Warwick and kingmaker.'" Dumas Malone, ed., Dictionary of American Biography, Vol. XX (New York: Charles Scribner s Sons, 1934), 659-660.

harmonious" and thanked his staff physicians, Dr. A. A. Padgett in 1854, and Dr. H. H. Bethshares in 1855, as well as Mr. and Mrs. Chatfield, for their services.

He added that he had spent a considerable amount of his own time supervising construction, and regretted that the noise from the work going on had made it impossible to "secure the tranquilizing influences of quiet and seclusion, so necessary to calm the excitement of this unfortunate class of patients."[40] He did not mention the arrival of an infant son in his own household on July 8, 1855, to join the sister who had also been born on the hospital grounds in 1853, a joyful event which had done little to improve his own quiet and seclusion.

Appended was the report of the architect, Major Heiman, who acknowledged his indebtedness to Dr. Cheatham and Miss Dorothea L. Dix, who had continued to maintain an active interest in the project, for valuable information relating to the construction of lunatic asylums. He noted that the main building should be faced with stone, want of funds having prevented it from being done at the time of construction, and that all exterior walls should be painted. The right wing lacked the whole interior finish, including the laying of the floors, and the plumbing for both wings, as well as air ducts, cisterns, and sewerage were "yet to be done to make the establishment what it is intended to be."[41]

In the Third Biennial Reports of 1859 Mr. Cockrill noted the purchase of 200 additional acres of land adjoining the original tract from James P. Johnson for $20,000, so that the state farm now contained 455 acres fronting on the Murfreesboro turnpike. The trustees were now satisfied that their building "is the best arranged, and combines more advantages than any other in the country of the same cost," and noted that other states had made large appropriations to erect asylums for the insane.[42]

A new treasurer, G. C. Torbett, reported receipts of $131,555.65 and disbursements in the same amount for the two-year period. Mr.

---

[40] Ibid., 45-47.
[41] Ibid., 51, 53-54.
[42] <u>Third Biennial Reports of the Trustees, Treasurer, Architect, and the Physician and Superintendent of the Tennessee Hospital for the Insane</u> (Nashville: G. C. Torbett & Co., 1857), 6-7.

Heiman gave his final report, noting that construction for the entire project had not exceeded $180,000, the excess of about $5,000 over his original estimate of $175,000 being a result of the rise in cost of materials and labor. He gave Dr. Cheatham "much credit for the saving of additional expenditures, by having a good deal of work done by the labor of some of the inmates of the establishment." He recommended some additional work, including the erection of a porter's lodge and iron gates which he had designed for the entrance, as well as stone facing and painting which he had recommended in the last report. He spoke admiringly of the green and propagating houses erected "in fine taste" by the superintendent, and closed his report "tendering to the Board of Trustees, and Dr. Cheatham, my heartfelt thanks for the efficient and courteous manner in which they have sustained me in my arduous duties."[43]

Dr. Cheatham reported that, of the 69 patients discharged during the two-year period, 28 were restored; 158 patients were under treatment at the date of his report, October 1, 1857. He also included various tables relating to the patients, and noted that the statistics of insanity indicate an 80 per cent recovery rate if treatment is resorted to in the early stages of the disease. He therefore called upon the press to enlighten the public about the kind treatment being given inmates of the hospital. He also called upon the public not to deceive patients about where they were being taken--"Better, far better, to force him to go against his will than to deceive him," Cheatham admonished.

To refute popular misconceptions, Cheatham described the amazed expression of someone being introduced to a well-administered modern hospital for the insane:

> His eyes and ears are painfully on the qui vive for unearthly screams and all the horrific paraphernalia of a dungeon. Judge of his astonishment when he perceives a large number of orderly ladies decently dressed; some engaged quietly in knitting or embroidery, some reading, and perhaps one at the piano eliciting exquisite tones, accompanied by the sweetest of voices; while another, absorbed in the music, is hanging over

---

[43] Ibid., 12 – 19.

the instrument and quietly turning the leaves of the music book for her friend. He passes to the male wards, half diposed [sic] to believe this an innocent trick played upon him by the Superintendent. Here he sees a large number of cleanly shaved and well dressed gentlemen--here are half a dozen round a billiard table; that young gentleman facing the window is discoursing sweet sounds upon a flute; another, no less skilled in music, is drawing delicious harmony from a violin; many are quietly devouring the morning papers, just arrived, while others are lost in works of history, biography, and fiction.

Continuing his project of educating the legislators and others about the latest principles of mental health, Cheatham included an excerpt from Dr. Brigham's Reports to the New York State Asylum at Utica, commenting on the tendency for a predisposition to insanity to be hereditary. Cheatham again admonished the legislature about the problem of allowing the institution to become custodial by failing to require counties to make bond for incurable cases. Again he gave an impressive farm report; this time the work was credited to four black men, assisted by the patients and their attendants and, in 1857, also by two black boys.

To the list of amusements he proudly announced the addition of an extensive greenhouse, well stocked with both native and exotic flowers and shrubs. It was, he wrote, "a most pleasing resort for the patients," reflecting that "few products of nature or art exercise so beguiling and soothing an influence upon an over-excited mind as flowers."

He thanked Hon. Charles Ready, Cheatham's father-in-law who was then serving a term in Washington as a U.S. Congressman, for seeds from the U.S. Patent Office and for important public documents. Hon. F. K. Zollicoffer had sent the same, and thanks went also to Miss Henrietta Cockrill and Mrs. John R. Wilson, each for a fine camellia for the greenhouse, and to Mrs. Thomas Washington for shrubs and flowers.

H. H. Bethshares, M. D., continued as assistant physician. Mr. Chatfield had retired with Mrs. Chatfield, both returning to their friends in New York. His place as steward had been taken by Thomas

Farmer, Esq., of Springfield, who was performing this duty most ably. And, since the departure of Mrs. Chatfield, Mrs. Cheatham had herself "assumed and discharged the duties of the office of matron."[44]

This amazing commitment on the part of Mrs. Cheatham, who was never in robust health, deserves some comment. As Dr. Cheatham indicated through his efforts to dispel some of the popular misconceptions about insanity, there was a stigma attached to mental illness, one that exists even today. Yet it was very much in the tradition of the Cheatham and Ready families to perform public service, and it is probably in that spirit, combined with a very deep personal commitment to her husband's work, that Mrs. Cheatham undertook this responsibility.

On January 14, 1859, Dr. Cheatham wrote Miss Dix to thank her for books, lanterns, stereoscopes, and a rocking boat which she had sent to the hospital to amuse the patients. She had also sent pictures which would soon be framed and distributed throughout the wards. Dr. Cheatham was pleased with their recent success in restoring patients to their normal lives. "As we advance & understand the specialty more, the greater the success which attends our efforts," he commented. He was pleased, too, over the acquisition of "two excellent white girls" as attendants on the female wards. "Our attendants now will, I think, compare favorably with many institutions, if not with the best in the country," he told Miss Dix. "We now have eighty female patients; & I know they are all made comfortable, & as well attended as in any institution in the country."[45]

He wrote again on February 10, thanking Miss Dix for a package of bulbs and expressing surprise that his last letters had not reached her. He discussed a couple of patients, commenting

> the longer I remain here & the more experience I have in the management of cases of mental disease, of course, enables me to accomplish more. I love the specialty; & if let alone by politicians would devote my life to it. But when the demagogues of the country, such men as Senator Johnson, are all the time

---

[44] Ibid., 27-51
[45] William A. Cheatham to Dorothea L. Dix, 14 January 1859, Houghton Library of Harvard University.

endeavoring to crush out every one who will not subscribe to their peculiar views, I confess that I feel like throwing up the position; & resuming a profession which I practiced before coming here with success.[46]

The Fourth Biennial Report, submitted on October 1, 1859, opened with the report of S. R. Cockrill, who enumerated significant improvements on roads, pavements, and walks. The road from the pike, 500 yards long, had been excavated about two feet, filled with stone, and finished off with gravel. Some 5,600 feet of stone curbing had been set on roads and walks, and more than 200,000 brick had been laid in pavements. A paved road had been laid to the rear· of the building, and a large brick smokehouse had been built to preserve supplies.

Cockrill noted that Dr. W. A. Cheatham had recently been re-elected by a unanimous vote of the board to another 8-year term. He gave to Dr. Cheatham much of the credit of the institution's "high position among similar institutions of the nation." The Tennessee Hospital for the Insane had even been written up in a Philadelphia periodical, which Cockrill cited:

> "The Doctor being an ardent horticulturist, has shown good taste in laying out the grounds, with an eye to landscape beauty and general picturesque effect. Insanity, the greatest affliction which can befall humanity, is here divested of all the horrors of treatment suffered under the old system. Kindness, quietude, and innocent amusements are the principal aids on which the doctor depends, for the relief and cure of his unfortunate patients, and one of the most efficient auxiliaries, is exercise in the beautiful and extensive pleasure grounds which surround and adorn the buildings."

Cockrill lauded the hospital for its "cleanliness, neatness, and good order." He added that the Trustees had encouraged the

---

[46] William A. Cheatham to Dorothea L. Dix, 10 February 1859, Houghton Library of Harvard University. A reference to former governor Andrew Johnson, elected U.S. Senator in 1857. Johnson, a Democrat, was violently opposed to the Whig power structure of which Cheatham was a member.

superintendent in his inclination "to embrace all improvements in agriculture, horticulture and domestic economy in the management of the farm," believing that would lead to higher production. When Mr. Underwood, who was apparently filling the position of gardener, brought his collection from the institution's greenhouses to the floral exhibition at the State Fair, several citizens had refused to compete. "He had no advantage except skill and attention," Cockrill insisted, "as we have made very small appropriations to these ornamental branches." He talked even of turning the project into a model farm, from which seeds and grains could be sent forth "to ornament and improve the country."

Even though the project was so well established, some improvements remained to be done: the grading of a road to a point on the Nashville and Chattanooga Railroad, to obtain coal for the use of the institution; conversion from candles and oil to gas for lighting; and a better water supply.[47]

A new treasurer, W. F. M'Gregor, reported receipts and disbursements each totaling $104,850.81,[48] almost $27,000 less than

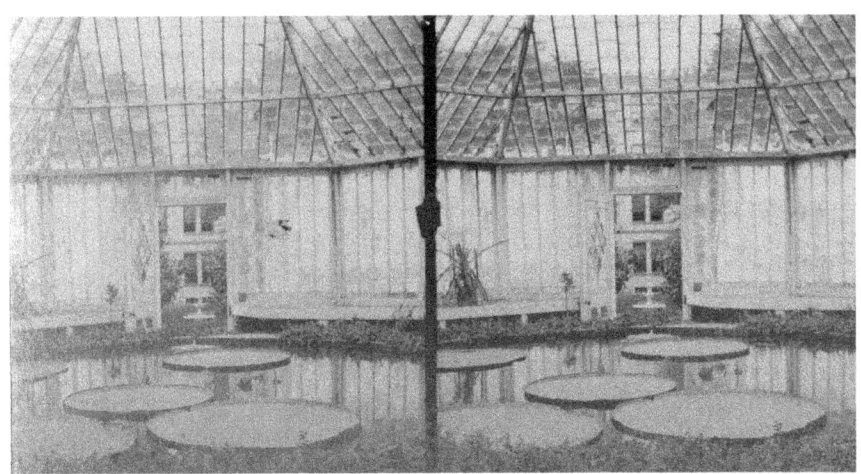

Stereoview of the Insane Asylum Greenhouse, including giant water lilies, by C. C. Giers. C. 1884. Courtesy of the Tennessee State Library and Archives.

---

[47] Fourth Biennial Reports of the Trustees, Treasurer, and the Superintendent and Physician of the Tennessee Hospital for the Insane (Nashville: E.G. Eastman & co., 1859), 5-14.
[48] Ibid., 19-20

the previous report, which must have been a relief to the legislators and probably indicated the level of operations they could expect in the future. Unquestionably it had been an expensive project; but it had brought great renown to the state, for which Dr. Cheatham was largely responsible.

Obviously moral treatment was expensive, and superintendents were categorically "opposed to all budget-cutting, believing it could lead only to the lowering of the quality of food and facilities for work and recreation, and reducing the number of staff." Superintendents realized also that the selection and training of attendants was essential to good treatment. Another important factor was the selection of a competent, active, and influential board of trustees.[49]

Cheatham had begun his superintendency with the assistance of Mr. and Mrs. Cyrus Chatfield, formerly steward and matron at the New York State asylum at Utica, New York, where they had served under Amariah Brigham.[50] They were initially a major asset in the training of competent staff. Cheatham had also begun his tenure with a distinguished board of trustees, presided over by Sterling R. Cockrill, who remained with him to the end. The support of his trustees, combined with Cheatham's own distinguished reputation and polished manner, was a significant factor in his ability to secure appropriations from the legislature and donations from private sources. The only instance where Cheatham encountered difficulties with the legislature was over the expense of administering the institution; but when an investigating committee inquired of Miss Dix whether the expenditures were excessive, "her reply was, that in this respect, as in all others, the institution compared most favorably with similar institutions."[51]

Since the last report, Dr. Cheatham recounted, 187 new patients had been admitted; 134 had been discharged or died, leaving 211 patients under treatment. Of the 134 discharged, 67 had been restored to health. He again included various tables interspersed with commentary. The farm yield was very high for 1858 and 1859; pork had

---

[49] Caplan, 33
[50] Reports (1853), 34
[51] House Journal of the First Session of the 33rd General Assembly of the State of Tennessee, Convened at Nashville October 1859 (Nashville: E. G. Eastman, & Co., 1859), 783.

become a major product, with not less than 12,000 pounds raised and currently being fattened in 1859. That year the farm force was composed of the farmer, two black men, three black boys, and the patients and their attendants. For the last fifteen months a tailor had been regularly employed who had, assisted by the female patients, made all their dresses. They continued to make quilts, hem linen, and assist in the wards, dining rooms, and ironing rooms.

Additional amusements included magic lanterns and stereoscopes, parties and concerts, 300 volumes added to the libraries in the wards, and 300 framed pictures hung in the wards. Miss Dorothea L. Dix, who spent a week in the institution in July of 1858, provided the pictures and selected the books, magic lanterns, and stereoscopes. "From its inception in her own benevolent mind to the present, she has taken a lively interest in its development," Dr. Cheatham wrote, "and her visit, while seemingly pleasant to her, was peculiarly gratifying to all connected with the establishment."

He noted also that the greenhouses had been greatly enlarged, furnishing a greater variety of plants and enabling them to provide fresh flowers for all the wards. Nothing, he felt, was more soothing to the diseased mind than flowers, and the greenhouses were a favorite retreat for patients who were able to take outdoor exercise, as were the rustic seats arranged on the grounds near the building.

To Mrs. Francis B. Fogg, through Miss Dix, they were indebted for an organ; to Mrs. General Jefferson Davis, of Hurricane, Mississippi, for shrubs; and to Hon. F. K. Zollicoffer, Hon. Charles Ready, and Hon. A. O. P. Nicholson[52] for public documents and seeds from the Patent Office.

He expressed particular thanks to Sterling R. Cockrill, the Chairman of the Board of Trustees, for his service of the last ten years,

---

[52] Alfred Osborne Pope Nicholson (1808-1876) was editor of the Washington Daily Union and public printer to the House of Representatives. In 1857 he was elected to succeed John Bell upon the expiration of his senatorial term in 1859. Nicholson was expelled from the Senate on July 11, 1861, for supporting the Confederacy. After the Civil War he served as Chief Justice of the Tennessee Supreme Court (1870-1876). A graduate of the University of North Carolina in 1827, he afterwards attended lectures in Jefferson Medical College in Philadelphia, but never practiced medicine. Dumas Malone, ed., Dictionary of American Biography, Vol. XIII (New York: Charles Scribner's Sons, 1934), 498.

his time given to the institution "without fee or reward." In conclusion, Dr. Cheatham expressed satisfaction with the work that had been done, all remaining "as perfect as science and art could secure, with the result "that our native State can boast of an institution which will compare favorably with any State institution in the United States."[53]

On November 25, 1859, Dr. Cheatham received a letter from Miss Dix, which he answered on December 2nd. "Well, I am expected to remain here another eight years," he announced in a satisfied tone. "On the 1st day of October last the board of Trustees met here, reelected me unanimously, passed a very complementary resolution, and adjourned." Plans were afoot to build an addition to the institution on an adjoining farm. "Since your visit we have improved the place considerably," he continued. "I think you will see something to admire." He was happy to add that Mrs. Cheatham's health was better than it had been for years. He concluded by asking Miss Dix to help in procuring the services of Miss Minerva Mendenhall, who had been the matron at Raleigh, to replace Miss Chatfield. He thus ended the year on a satisfied note, gratified at what had been accomplished, newly reappointed as superintendent, and in the mood to prosecute "this good work with more energy than ever."[54]

Stereoview of the lake at the Insane Asylum. C. 1884.
Courtesy of the Tennessee State Library and Archives

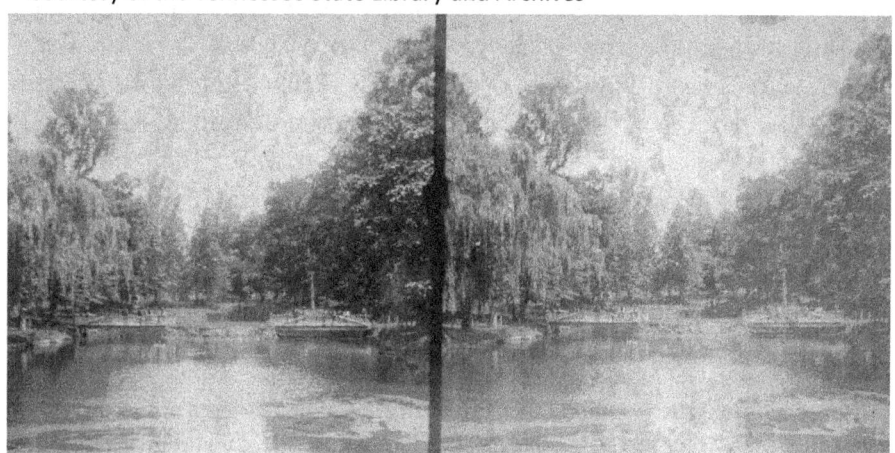

---

[53] Fourth Biennial Reports (1859), 21-48.
[54] William A. Cheatham to Dorothea L. Dix, 2 December 1859, Houghton Library of Harvard University.

CHAPTER 4
AN EVALUATION OF DR. CHEATHAM AND THE TENNESSEE HOSPITAL FOR THE INSANE, 1852-1862

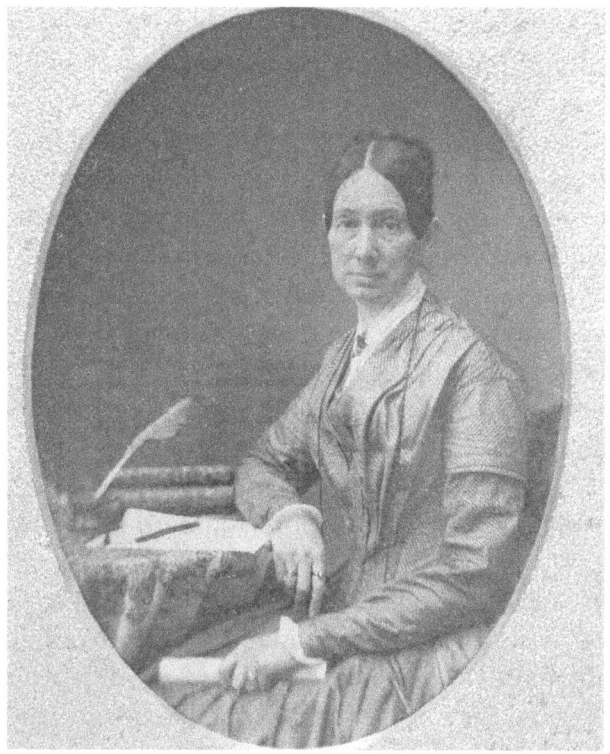

Dorothea Lynde Dix (1802-1887), c. 1849.
Courtesy of the National Portrait Gallery.

In July of 1858, when Dorothea L. Dix visited the Tennessee Hospital for the Insane, she said to Sterling R. Cockrill, President of the Board of Trustees, "' There are but few institutions anywhere, superior to the Tennessee Hospital for the Insane,' and none equal to it in the south-west." Cockrill pointed out that Miss Dix knew by personal observation what was being done in similar hospitals all over the world; and furthermore, that she was "intelligent, truthful, and a lady in every sense of the word."[1] If Miss Dix can be taken at her word, the Tennessee Hospital for the Insane and its superintendent, Dr. William Archer Cheatham, can claim leadership in the Southwest and equal rank with most institutions for the mentally ill in mid-nineteenth century America.

Some would find this too ambitious a claim. Paul R. Dokecki and Janice D. Mashburn in <u>Beyond the Asylum: The History of Mental Handicap Policy in Tennessee: 1796-1984</u> write as follows:

> Dix's compliment is somewhat puzzling, since it is doubtful that the Tennessee institution ever compared favorably with some of the better funded Eastern corporate and state hospitals. In fact, most authorities note that the Southern hospitals, even at their best, were never equal to their Northern counterparts. Perhaps Dix was pleased to see that the state had made at least minimal progress in providing for its insane and she wanted to acknowledge the fact that the legislature had followed the recommendations she had made a decade earlier.[2]

Most authorities tend to ignore southern hospitals, and there are in fact not many comparisons between northern and southern hospitals; but when the South is singled out, the suggestion is rather that the South tended to lag behind the North. Norman Dain, for example, comments in a footnote that moral treatment in the South often lagged behind that in the North, although he does not document this statement.[3] However, to lag behind does not necessarily imply a failure to measure up eventually to a given standard of performance. There is no reason to think that a Tennessee institution could categorically fail to compare favorably with the better eastern

---

[1] <u>Fourth Biennial Reports of the Trustees, Treasurer, and the Superintendent and Physician of the Tennessee Hospital for the Insane</u> (Nashville: E. G. Eastman & Co., 1859), 12.
[2] Paul R, Dokecki and Janice D. Mashburn, <u>Beyond the Asylum: The History of Mental Handicap Policy in Tennessee, 1796-1948</u> (Nashville: Tennessee Department of Mental Health and Retardation, 1984), 20.
[3] Norman Dain, <u>Concepts of Insanity in the United States, 1789- 1865</u> (New Brunswick, NJ: Rutgers University Press, 1964), 55.

institutions. Nor was it necessarily less well funded, nor was Miss Dix necessarily insincere in her praise of the institution.

Dr. William A. Cheatham and the Tennessee Hospital for the Insane must be evaluated first, in the context of the reform movement in Tennessee and the rest of the nation; second, in terms of the program of moral treatment which was the hallmark of psychiatry in the first half of the nineteenth century; and third, in terms of the professional recognition accorded Cheatham and his institution. One can then state with more certainty just where Tennessee and its superintendent stood in the period 1852-1862 in relation to other institutions dealing exclusively with the mentally ill.

The reform era in Tennessee, extending approximately from the 1820s through the 1840s, was an humanitarian outgrowth of the Enlightenment and the Great Awakening; in Tennessee, during the 1830s and 1840s, the movement focused on the plight of the insane.[4] During the summer of 1836, Dr. James Overton visited institutions in the Northeast, where he was impressed by the Puritan and Quaker retreats in Connecticut and Pennsylvania. The following year, in 1837, Governor Newton Cannon successfully requested of the legislature funds to build an asylum. In 1840 Tennessee's first asylum began operation with Dr. John Kelley as superintendent. It accommodated fewer than 60 patients, however, out of nearly 800 pauper lunatics residing in Tennessee.[5]

In April of 1846 Dorothea L. Dix, noted reformer and advocate of state-supported hospitals for the mentally ill, visited Tennessee to inspect its facilities and treatment for the care of the mentally ill, which she pronounced totally inadequate. On December 14, 1847, she

---

[4] E. Bruce Thompson, "Reforms in the Care of the Insane in Tennessee, 1830-1850," Tennessee Historical Quarterly III (4) (December 1944): 319. Reforms also included a school for the blind in Nashville (1842) and a school for the deaf in Knoxville (1844).

[5] Ibid., 324-325. Dr. James Overton was a member of a prominent Middle Tennessee family. Like other physicians of his day, he had no particular training in mental illness, generally called insanity in the nineteenth century. But his visit to the Northeast is an indication that Tennesseans wished to educate themselves about treatment at the leading institutions.

delivered a memorial to the legislature, requesting funds to build a much larger, modern facility in a rural setting.[6]

On February 5, 1848, the legislature passed a bill to establish a hospital embodying her ideas: "the bill, on the whole, was one of the most enlightened pieces of legislation emanating from the Tennessee legislature prior to the Civil War."[7] The commissioners purchased a 255-acre farm, property of the late Henry Dickinson, on the Murfreesboro Road six miles south of Nashville.[8] Dr. John S. Young, who was appointed superintendent, visited northern asylums to formulate plans based on the New Jersey Hospital for the Insane; the Butler Asylum in Rhode Island, erected under the supervision of Dr. Luther Bell of the McLean Asylum in Massachusetts, and incorporating features of it; and the Bloomingdale Hospital in New York.[9]

Upon the recommendation of Dr. Young, Major Adolphus Heiman was selected as architect and construction began in the fall of 1848.[10] The hospital was nearing completion in October of 1852,[11] but it was still not completely finished. Nevertheless, in April of 1852 the new superintendent, Dr. William A. Cheatham, supervised the removal of the patients from the old institution to the new.[12]

This was Tennessee's response to the reform movement that was not peculiar to the state, nor to the South; nor was the movement confined to the insane: the temperance crusade in the 1840s and 1850s also cut across state and sectional boundaries. Other northern reforms,

---

[6] Helen E. Marshall, Dorothea Dix, Forgotten Samaritan (Chapel Hill: University of North Carolina Press, 1937), 113, 116; Dorothy Clarke Wilson, Stranger and Traveler: The Story of Dorothea Dix, American Reformer (Boston: Little, Brown and Company, 1975), 167.
[7] Thompson, 333.
[8] W. K. Bowling, M.D., and Paul F. Eve, M.D., eds., The Nashville Journal of Medicine and Surgery V (October 1851): 299; Frank Luton, M.D., and Charles E. Goshen, M.D., "A Brief History of Tennessee Psychiatry," Journal of the Tennessee Medical Association 65 (8) (August 1862): 711.
[9] Bowling, 299.
[10] Luton, 711; Thompson, 334.
[11] Bowling, 299.
[12] Reports of the Trustees, Treasurer and Physician of the Tennessee Hospital for the Insane, Transmitted to the Legislature on the Sixth November, 1853 (Nashville: Union and American Steam Press, 1853): 15.

however, such as women's rights and anti-slavery, made little or no headway in the South. Still, "something besides Southern provincialism and self-consciousness characterized this section in the decade before the Civil War," wrote Avery O. Craven in <u>The Growth of Southern Nationalism, 1848-1861</u>. "There were likenesses between the North and South as well as differences."[13] Seen in this light, the reform movement on behalf of the insane gains significance as a unifying, nationalizing force in opposition to growing sectional division in other areas. A major significance of Dorothea L. Dix's crusade is that it did not recognize state, regional, or even national boundaries.

Clement A. Eaton, discussing the reform movement in <u>A History of the Old South</u>, suggests that the growth of humanitarianism was "closely associated with the religiousness of the South."[14] He points to considerable progress by 1860, not only in the establishment of hospitals for the insane in all states except Florida before the outbreak of the Civil War, but also in the gradual abolition of cock-fighting, gouging, and dueling, as well as the temperance movement, some humanization of criminal codes and procedures, and prison reform.[15]

Nor does he relinquish leadership to the North. Unquestionably northern institutions were leaders in new methods of treatment, hospital planning, and administration; but a case can be made for southern leadership in establishing the precedent of state responsibility for the care of the mentally ill. Eaton points out that the first state hospital for the insane was established by the Virginia legislature at Williamsburg in 1773; that Kentucky established the second state institution exclusively for the insane in 1824; and that South Carolina, in 1828, was the third state to provide an asylum.[16]

Tennessee's program for the mentally ill incorporated the most advanced theories of the period. A communal atmosphere prevailed at the Tennessee Hospital for the Insane, as elsewhere in moral treatment

---

[13] Avery O. Craven, <u>The Growth of Southern Nationalism, 1848- 1861</u>, Vol. VI of <u>A History of the South</u>, Wendell Holmes Stephenson and E. Merton Coulter, eds. (Baton Rouge: Louisiana State University Press, 1953), 164.
[14] Clement Eaton, <u>A History of the Old South</u> (New York: The Macmillan Company, 1949), 496.
[15] Ibid., 497-499.
[16] Ibid., 498-499.

programs. Patients were encouraged to discuss their problems with one another, and work was usually done in groups. Diversions and amusements, which included games, reading, carriage rides, walks, dances, religious services, lectures, and recitations, were designed "to inculcate normal cultural values and modalities so that the individual could return to society better able to cope with its demands."[17]

At the 15th annual meeting of the AMSAII, Dr. Cheatham had stated that he "deemed amusements among the most effective curative agents, and in his institution there was everything that could possibly be obtained for that purpose. In the winter months there were frequent exhibitions of the magic lantern, concerts, social parties, and dancing. A great deal of time was devoted to the cultivation of flowers, for which the section of country offered peculiar facilities. His patients were for the most part agricultural in their habits."[18]

Moral treatment, although impractical by today's standards and naive by the standards of twentieth century psychiatry, represents a progressive movement "that included a kind of milieu therapy for patients and a deep involvement of practitioners in the affairs of the lay community. The system also developed a number of assumptions that molded, with mixed results, the course of subsequent professional development."[19] Some of its characteristics were institutionalization; partnership between laymen and professionals; legislation governing insanity; optimism, that is, the expectation that insanity could be cured; and the imposition of the medical model on the care of the insane.[20] Tennessee's program implemented all of these.

The partnership with the lay community had mixed results. Laymen, especially legislators, were typically involved in the establishment and administration of mental hospitals. This partnership was successful when it involved "enlightened and generous patrons and enthusiastic, effective superintendents," as in the case of Dr. William A. Cheatham and his supporters. But in most cases friction arose over laws

---

[17] Ruth B. Caplan, Psychiatry and the Community in Nineteenth Century America (New York: Basic Books, Inc., 1969), 38.
[18] American Journal of Insanity XVII (July 1860), 69.
[19] Caplan, 47.
[20] Ibid., 48-49.

and regulations; and when superintendents lost control over admissions, overcrowding and financial problems resulted. Overburdened superintendents began to lose touch with their patients and the community as they spent more and more time lobbying for funds.[21]

In their efforts to enlist public support, the superintendents oversold moral treatment, with a resulting disillusionment. But it had a lasting impact on the profession in that "it attracted active, idealistic men, confident of their eventual mastery of insanity. Their personalities and programs hence differed significantly from those of later practitioners who would be recruited to a more hopeless and static profession."[22]

Inevitably, perhaps, the program of moral treatment at the Tennessee Hospital for the Insane would have gone the way of all other institutions by the 1870s, which ushered in an era of pessimism and custodial care[23] that lasted well into the twentieth century. But Dr. Cheatham's reign as superintendent of the Tennessee Hospital for the Insane was ended by political intervention when he was removed from office by Andrew Johnson, Military Governor of the State of Tennessee, in July of 1862. As a member of the secessionist power structure and cousin of General B. F. Cheatham, Dr. William A. Cheatham was not acceptable to the Union occupation as superintendent of one of the state's major institutions. Thus he retired to private life and private practice; but he maintained his interest in the mentally ill and thereafter specialized in the practice of what we would today call psychiatry.

To evaluate his contribution, we must first turn to his contemporaries. Dr. W. K. Bowling, editor of the <u>Nashville Journal of Medicine and Surgery</u>, wrote, less than two years after Cheatham became superintendent, that he had been "ardent and indefatigable," achieving a "triumphant success [which] must be highly gratifying to

---

[21] Ibid., 63-65, 70, 86.
[22] Ibid., 89-90.
[23] Whereas moral treatment, with its emphasis on curability, was an expression of optimism, the gradual lapse into custodial care reflected the pessimistic attitude that mental illness could not be cured.

himself, his friends, and the state generally." Dr. Bowling added that "Dr. Cheatham is peculiarly fitted by high professional qualifications, polished softness of manner, and sleepless energy of character, for this high and responsible position."[24]

Bowling's praise remained constant. "The general health of the institution has been excellent," he wrote in 1860. "It has been fortunate in the excellence of its managers and physicians, and is a credit and honor to our state." He added that the superintendent is appreciated by the trustees, "who have shown their good judgement in reelecting him."[25]

There is no question that William A. Cheatham had both high standing and credibility among his contemporaries in Tennessee, and it is also clear that he was warmly supported by Dorothea L. Dix, who kept in close touch with the Tennessee Hospital for the Insane, which she had helped create. But there is still the question of whether Miss Dix exaggerated when she said there were few institutions superior to the Tennessee Hospital for the Insane, and none equal to it in the Southwest. That can be fully appraised, insofar as possible given the information available today, only by the application of some national standard. The only source that would meet that criterion is the American Journal of Insanity, the official publication of Dr. Cheatham's professional organization, the AMSAII, with particular attention to the reports of the annual meetings.

Dr. William A. Cheatham attended the ninth annual meeting of the AMSAII at the Smithsonian Institution in Washington, D.C., on Tuesday, May 9, 1854, in the company of such illustrious practitioners and pioneers in the field of mental illness as Dr. Luther V. Bell, of the McLean Asylum; Dr. Issac Ray, of Butler Hospital; Dr. Francis T. Stribling, of the Western Asylum in Staunton, Virginia; Dr. Thomas S. Kirkbride, of the Pennsylvania Hospital for the Insane; Dr. John Curven, of the Pennsylvania State Lunatic Asylum; Dr. Edward Jarvis, representing a private asylum in Dorchester, Massachusetts; and Dr. William M. Awl, late of the Ohio State Lunatic Asylum. Of the twenty-two superintendents, only Dr. Cheatham, Dr. Stribling, and Dr. Edward

---

[24] Bowling, VI (June 1854), 107.
[25] Ibid., XVIII (1860), 138.

C. Fisher of the Insane Asylum in Raleigh, North Carolina, represented southern states.[26]

The superintendents met through May 12, spending that morning at Mount Vernon. At the 6 p.m. adjournment, they thanked Lieutenant Matthew Fontaine Maury of the U.S. Observatory and Professor Alexander Dallas Bache of the Coast Survey for opening their establishments; Robert McClelland, Secretary of the Interior, for accompanying them to the U.S. Hospital for the Insane; and W. W. Corcoran, Esquire, for opening his private gallery of art to them. During the week they had held seminars on various subjects, the more prominent among them giving papers and indulging in heated discussion.[27] Newcomers like Dr. Cheatham were conspicuously quiet. However, just the fact of his presence was significant; he had benefited from the opportunity to know and become known by the leaders of the rising psychiatric profession in the United States, to become exposed to their ideas, and to represent his state at a national meeting.

Dr. Cheatham did not attend the 10th annual meeting in 1855, which was held in Boston; but he was present at the 11th annual meeting in Cincinnati, Ohio, which began on Monday, May 19, 1856. At this meeting he was the only representative of the states which later seceded from the Union. He did not participate in the discussion following several papers, but it was on his motion that the association adjourned to meet in New York City in May of 1857.[28]

At the 12th annual meeting only Dr. Fisher of North Carolina attended from the southern states; and only Dr. Thomas F. Green, representing the state lunatic asylum at Milledgeville, Georgia, attended from the South when the superintendents met in Quebec for their 13th annual meeting in 1858. But in 1859, on Tuesday, May 17, Dr. Cheatham was present for the 14th annual meeting in Lexington, Kentucky, as were superintendents representing state asylums in Mississippi and Louisiana.[29]

Following a paper on the use of forced tube feeding for patients who refused to eat, Dr. Cheatham demonstrated his own use of innate

---

[26] American Journal of Insanity XI (July 1854), 37-38.
[27] Ibid., 55.
[28] American Journal of Insanity XII (July 1855), 39; XIII (July 1856), 82-88.
[29] Ibid., XVI (July 1857), 69; XV (July 1858), 77; XVI (July 1859), 42.

common sense in the resulting discussion. He told how "he had often compelled patients to eat who had been commanded by God to fast, by telling them that the Lord had also commanded him to make them eat."[30]

Dr. William A. Cheatham was the only representative of the southern states to attend the 15th annual meeting in Philadelphia on Monday, May 28, 1860. At this meeting he was appointed to the Committee on Resolutions, an assignment which indicates that he had begun to achieve a certain prestige within the AMSAII. He was much more outspoken than he had previously been at an annual meeting, commenting at length on dipsomania as a disease related to alcoholism. He went so far as to state that he "could never have confidence in the entire reformation of anyone who had become the victim of an indulgence" and "would not consider them safe if a period of thirty years had elapsed."[31]

After Dr. McFarland had read a paper on attendants, Dr. Cheatham commented that black girls owned by the asylum were the best attendants on his female wards, being "more kind and faithful, and more acceptable to those of whom they had the care, than any white person they could employ." Dr. Kirkbride, who probably considered this a touchy subject, responded that the "fact of nationality" was hardly worth considering, giving as an example the excellent attendants he had found among the Irish, "a class of whom most of the members had related an unfavorable experience, in their institutions."[32]

On the following morning, at the request of association president Dr. Andrew McFarland of Illinois, Dr. Cheatham took the chair,[33] another mark of prestige and acceptance for the superintendent from Tennessee. As if sensing encouragement, Dr. Cheatham again contributed to discussion, this time citing his views on recreation, quoted earlier. This meeting was both the culmination and the termination of his career in that elite group, the AMSAII, an organization which itself was beginning the transformation from a

---

[30] Ibid., 68.
[31] Ibid., XVII (July 1860), 5.
[32] Ibid., 60.
[33] Ibid., 61.

pioneering role representing progressive reform to a "narrow intellectual and institutional posture."[34]

Dr. Cheatham's repeated attendance at meetings and his acceptance by the leadership of the AMSAII appears to support Miss Dix's contention that no program in the Southwest was equal, in professional status at least, to that of the Tennessee Hospital for the Insane. It also indicates that William A. Cheatham had achieved professional equality for himself and his institution among other, almost exclusively northern, superintendents and institutions.

The testimony of those closer to home is clearly supportive of this interpretation. Dr. Bowling, editor of the state's leading medical journal, consistently praised Dr. Cheatham's capabilities and achievements. Sterling Cockrill and other trustees of the hospital unanimously elected Dr. Cheatham to a second eight-year term in 1859. At that time Mr. Cockrill gave to Dr. Cheatham much of the credit for the institution's "high position among similar institutions of the nation," citing a laudatory article from a Philadelphia periodical in addition to the high appraisal of Miss Dix.[35]

Tennessee was not the first in the nation, or in the South, to provide institutional care for the mentally ill. Nor was Dr. William A. Cheatham the only individual responsible for Tennessee's success in establishing a modern institution centered around a program of moral treatment. Many laid the groundwork and provided the support that created and sustained the Tennessee Hospital for the Insane. But Dr. Cheatham, selected by his peers to assume leadership of the institution from the outset, invested the ten most productive years of his professional life in creating a model program of moral treatment. He thereby achieved for himself and the Tennessee Hospital for the Insane a regional and even national reputation for excellence of which his fellow Tennesseans were justifiably proud.

---

[34] Charles E. Rosenberg, The Trial of the Assassin Guiteau: Psychiatry and Law in the Gilded Age (Chicago: University of Chicago Press, 1968), 61.
[35] Reports (1859), 10-11.

CHAPTER 5
DISRUPTION: THE IMPACT OF THE UNION OCCUPATION ON THE LIFE AND CAREER OF DR. CHEATHAM

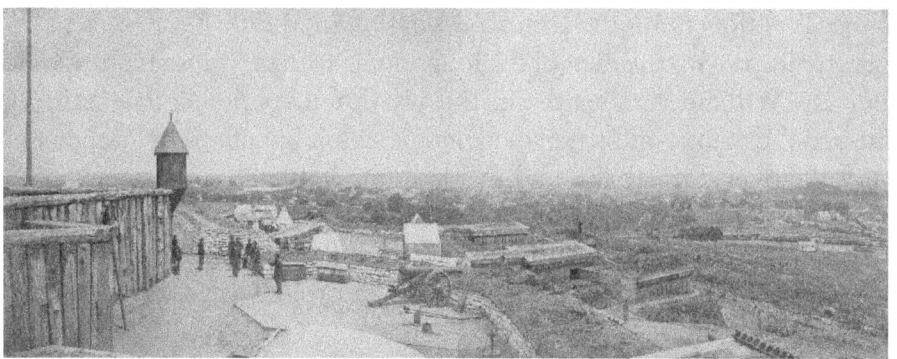

Fort Negley, Nashville, Tennessee. Taken in March of 1864 by George N. Barnard. Courtesy of the Library of Congress.

"It is one of the ironies of the Southern experience that in the very hour of the region's greatest public optimism and self-assurance, external and internal forces were conspiring to overturn the Southern world."[1] Indeed, the chain of events which transformed Middle Tennessee beginning in the spring of 1861 must have seemed like a conspiracy to Dr. William A. Cheatham, superintendent of the Tennessee Hospital for the Insane. His institution, the culmination of the reform movement which had swept Tennessee in the 1830s and 40s, was in itself an expression of public optimism. His self-assurance, based on ten years of impressive achievement, entitled him to claim equal standing with any hospital in the United States dealing exclusively with the mentally ill.

The Civil War affected both Dr. Cheatham and the Tennessee Hospital for the Insane. "The land and the people were not the only casualties of war," Stephen Ash has proposed. "The region's

---

[1] Stephen V. Ash, <u>Middle Tennessee Society Transformed, 1860-1870</u> (Baton Rouge: Louisiana State University Press, 1988), 64.

institutions, those inveterate manifestations of society's deepest convictions and loftiest achievements, also suffered in the years of turmoil following the invasion. . . ; but few escaped some disruption, and many sustained crippling and near-mortal wounds."[2] Among those institutions experiencing disruption was the Tennessee Hospital for the Insane, which suffered the depredations of troops from both armies moving along Murfreesboro Road, loss of state funds, and a change in superintendents. But the Union occupation of Middle Tennessee had a greater impact on the lives of the individuals who ran those institutions. For Dr. William A. Cheatham, the wartime experience dramatically altered the course of his personal and professional life. What happened to William A. Cheatham, and to his immediate and extended family, supports C. Vann Woodward's theory that the Civil War had devastating effects on Southern life, producing something akin to a revolution and unseating those who had controlled its government and institutions.[3]

An investigation of the war's impact on the life of Dr. Cheatham will indicate that the revolution was partly accidental, attributable to the fortunes of war; but it was primarily the result of a planned attempt by the occupying forces to destroy the leadership of the secessionist regime. Andrew Johnson, Military Governor of Tennessee, and also Union generals Don Carlos Buell, William S. Rosecrans, and Henry W. Halleck, represented these forces, which were ultimately successful.

Although Tennesseans voted to secede from the Union in a referendum on June 8, 1861, it was not until February 1862 that Middle Tennesseans actually confronted the reality of war. Albert Sidney Johnston, whom President Davis had appointed general commanding the Western Department of the Confederate States of America, had decided to protect Tennessee's northern border by fortifying Forts Henry and Donelson on the Tennessee and Cumberland rivers.

The reaction from Middle Tennesseans was decidedly apathetic, despite the fact that Nashville was a major supply base for the Confederacy and therefore an obvious military target. The forts were

---

[2] Ibid., 95.
[3] C. Vann Woodward, <u>Thinking Back: The Perils of Writing History</u> (Baton Rouge: Louisiana State University Press, 1986), 74.

not completed when Union troops, under General Ulysses S. Grant, attacked in early February.[4]

Shock waves swept through the South when Fort Donelson fell on February 16, 1862, but nowhere was the effect so great as in Nashville, now open to the enemy. The rumor that Fort Donelson had surrendered swept Nashville on Sunday, February 16, setting off

> a reign of terror and confusion. . ., the like of which was never witnessed in Nashville. Men and women were to be seen running to and fro in every portion of the city, and large numbers were hastening with their valuables to the several railroad depots, or escaping in private conveyances to some place of fancied security in the country.   The hire of private conveyances was put up to fabulous prices, and it was only the wealthy that could enjoy the luxury of a ride on that day. Large numbers, in their eagerness to escape from the city, left on foot carrying with them such articles as they wished to preserve . . . and, of course, these must necessarily have been few.[5]

At least 1,000 left the city, including Governor Isham Harris and the legislature and such prominent individuals as Joseph A. S. Acklen, who departed for his wife's Louisiana plantations. Mrs. Acklen was among those who sent valuables to Sarah Childress Polk, the widow of former President James K. Polk, for safekeeping.[6]

On that Sunday, General A. S. Johnston's army passed through Nashville on its retreat to Murfreesboro, having marched thirty miles in one day in rain, snow, and ice. "Some of the last units to arrive camped overnight along the turnpike from near Mill Creek to the insane asylum," wrote Confederate officer Charles R. Mott, Jr., in his war

---

[4] Robert E. Corlew, Tennessee, A Short History, 2d ed. (Knoxville: The University of Tennessee Press, 1984), 293, 304-306.
[5] Stanley F. Horn, Tennessee's War, 1861-1865 (Nashville: Tennessee Civil War Centennial Commission, 1965), 61-62.
[6] Walter T. Durham, Nashville: The Occupied City (The First Seventeen Months-- February 16, 1862, to June 30, 1863) (Nashville: Tennessee Historical Society, 1985), 11-12, 18, 20.

journal. "The light of their campfires was clearly visible from Rutledge Hill in the city."[7]

The light of their fires would have been even more clearly visible to Dr. Cheatham and the inmates of the Tennessee Hospital for the Insane, which was set less than a quarter of a mile from Murfreesboro Road about six miles south of Nashville.   In fact, it is likely that the hospital had furnished wood for many of those fires, for the soldiers "had to cut down trees, burn fence rails, and take hay and corn in the neighborhoods surrounding the campsites."[8]

From the retreating army, Dr. Cheatham must have learned of the disaster at Forts Henry and Donelson, and the subsequent decision to abandon Nashville, with its rich store of supplies. On the following day, Monday, February 17, Generals John B. Floyd and Gideon Pillow arrived in Nashville by riverboat. Moments after his arrival, General Floyd assumed command of the city. Large crowds were swarming the warehouses where distribution of public stores had begun early that morning; but General Floyd "closed the stores to the public and announced that supplies, except those needed for hospitals, would be shipped south at once for use of the army."[9] By the morning of the 18th, however, there was a vast crowd nearly out of control at the quartermaster and commissary stores. When General N. B. Forrest rode in, General Floyd placed him in charge of the city and of the stores almost before he could dismount from his horse.[10]

In the interval, Dr. William A. Cheatham had come into Nashville to request supplies from General Floyd. When the governor and legislators had fled on Sunday, February 16, they took with them all funds for support of the institution. Dr. Cheatham was outraged and indignant when General Floyd, who "with a large quantity of Quartermaster and Commissary supplies in the city, that he could not take with him, and which were afterwards scattered in every direction,

---

[7] Ibid., 9.
[8] Ibid.
[9] Ibid., 22.
[10] Ibid., 32.

he, upon my application to him in person, at his headquarters in the St. Cloud Hotel, bade me begone, and that I could get nothing."[11]

The hospital was now without funds for food and clothing. These were supplied by private donations from Cheatham's friends M. A. Parrish, R. C. McNairy, Dr. John L. Cheatham, and James McLaughlin.[12] Under normal conditions, Dr. Cheatham might have been able to call on his brother, Nashville mayor Richard B. Cheatham, his cousin, Confederate general, B. F. Cheatham, or upon his wife's influential family in Murfreesboro. But the traditional network of support upon which he and others in Middle Tennessee leadership positions had once been able to depend was now disrupted by the Union occupation of Nashville.

Murfreesboro Road had now become a military thoroughfare upon which armies passed between Nashville and Chattanooga, with the result that the hospital became a conference site for generals on both sides. From the outset, the atmosphere at the hospital was charged with the tensions arising from war. Income from both the state and relatives of patients had dwindled to nothing, yet non-paying patients continued to be supported by the institution.

Cheatham reported as follows:

> The armies that had swept by or loitered in the neighborhood took whatever they needed or found untaken. The funds that had been provided for the institution disappeared with the retreating army and amid the prevailing excitement amounting almost to consternation, nothing more, if so much, could be expected of individuals than that each should take care of

---

[11] Report of William A. Cheatham dated Nashville, January 23, 1866, Appendix to Senate Journal, 1865-66: 226.

[12] Ibid. R. C. McNairy was a Nashville dry goods merchant whom General Forrest commended as one of several citizens assisting him with the evacuation of Nashville. Durham, Nashville, 44. Dr. John L. Cheatham (1832-1863) was Dr. W. A. Cheatham's first cousin and also the stepson of Dr. W. K. Bowling, with whom he practiced medicine until failing health compelled him to retire shortly before his death on September 29, 1863. Obsequies of John L. Cheatham, M. D. of Nashville, Tennessee, with an address by J.B. Ferguson (Nashville: John T. S. Fall, 1863). M. A. Parrish was a wholesale grocer and commission agent in Nashville.

himself, so that at times it has seemed to me almost a miracle that nearly 300 people, more than two- thirds of which [were] bereft of reason, could not only be held together but kept comfortable.

No employee abandoned his post, even though salaries were cut off.[13]

Almost prophetically, Federal spies and agents had reached Nashville ahead of the army. On February 25th the first sizeable contingent of Yankees arrived in Nashville.[14] The occupation was not immediately consolidated, however; on February 26th Confederate general W. J. Hardee sent Captain John Hunt Morgan with a few selected men into Nashville to sink the ferry-steamboat "Minnetonka," which the daring Morgan accomplished, afterwards fleeing towards Lebanon.[15] This, too, was prophetic of later events.

Nashville, in the words of Provost Judge John Fitch, "was a rebel city, occupied as conquered territory, and swarming with traitors, smugglers, and spies."[16] For a short time General Don Carlos Buell was in command of the city from his headquarters at the St. Cloud Hotel, so recently vacated by General Floyd. Despite the opposition of Buell, President Lincoln decided to appoint a military governor whose mission would be to return Tennessee and its citizens to the Union. On March 3, 1862, Lincoln named Andrew Johnson to the post, giving him the additional military rank of brigadier-general of volunteers. Johnson arrived in Nashville by train, in a boxcar, on the night of March 12.[17]

Meanwhile, on Sunday, March 9, John Hunt Morgan skirmished with Union troops on Franklin Pike. Later in the day, he obtained a pass from General Mitchell and went into Nashville, where he dined at the City Hotel.[18] There Morgan enjoyed a good dinner. More

---

[13] Ibid.
[14] Durham, Nashville, 40, 46.
[15] Ibid., 51.
[16] Horn, 124
[17] Clifton R. Hall, Andrew Johnson, Military Governor of Tennessee (Princeton, NJ: Princeton University Press, 1916), 19 ; Durham, Nashville, 55-59; LeRoy P. Graf and Ralph w. Haskins, eds., The Papers of Andrew Johnson, Vol. 5, 1861-62 (Knoxville: The University of Tennessee Press, 1969), xxxv.
[18] Durham, Nashville, 67

importantly, he demonstrated that Union forces clearly had failed to consolidate their hold on the city, where the sentiment of the white population was overwhelmingly secessionist.

Although Dr. William A. Cheatham was superintendent of the Tennessee Hospital for the Insane during both of Johnson's gubernatorial terms,[19] the two were not natural allies. William's brother, Edward S. Cheatham, representing Johnson's Know-Nothing opposition, was elected speaker of the senate in 1855.[20] In 1857, the legislature elected Governor Johnson to succeed J. C. Jones in the U. S. Senate. Four years later, in 1861, Johnson was the only U. S. Senator from a seceding state to retain his seat.[21]

Johnson biographer Clifton R. Hall wrote that "his greatest assets were a brilliant, incisive mind and an insatiable ambition; these proved decisive of his career. Breadth of view he never attained." Johnson, who was economically and culturally deprived in his youth, deeply resented those with wealth and social standing. This bitterness "grew upon him with years, poisoned his whole life, and impaired his character." His idea always was to advance the common man "at the expense of intrenched privilege," especially the slave-holding aristocracy. "If Johnson were a snake," said his rival, Governor Isham G. Harris, "he would lie in the grass to bite the heels of rich men's children."[22] Above all, Andrew Johnson hated a gentleman.

Johnson's appointment as military governor was universally unpopular. His opposition to slavery and secession, and his retention of his U. S. Senate seat after Tennessee seceded, alienated the Southern Democratic Party. His 1860 support of the Southern Democratic ticket had alienated the Unionists of East Tennessee, who also resented his antagonism to William G. Brownlow, a leader of that group. Furthermore, his devotion to the Democratic Party created opposition

---

[19] Corlew, 276. Andrew Johnson, born in 1808 in Raleigh, North Carolina, to a poor family, had no formal education. After settling in Greeneville, Tennessee, in 1826, Johnson opened a tailor shop. He became active in local politics. In 1835 and 1839 he won election to the state legislature and in 1841 to the state senate. Elected to Congress in 1843, he remained in Washington, D.C., until his election as governor of Tennessee in 1853 and again in 1855.
[20] Ibid., 280.
[21] Ibid., 282; Hall, 25.
[22] Hall, 20-22.

among northern Radicals and the national Republican administration. Finally, unpopularity was intrinsic in the very position he was sent to fill, because it had no precedent.[23]

The difficulties of the office fell into two categories, administrative and constitutional. Administratively, Johnson had to deal with three categories of constituents: loyalists, active secessionists, and neutrals. There were administrative clashes with Generals Buell and Halleck, whose armies were operating in the same area, and who "were certain to view with impatience and intolerance the projects of a civil officer whose very presence they disapproved."[24]

The constitutional validity of the office of military governor was questionable; among those who questioned it was Thaddeus Stevens. Johnson's unpopularity, combined with the administrative and constitutional weaknesses of the office, brought an outburst of plots against his life, kidnapping attempts, and hate mail.[25]

An added annoyance was the continuing presence of John Hunt Morgan, who lurked on the outskirts of Nashville. Morgan had many friends and supporters, including the Ready family of Murfreesboro.

On March 15, Alice Ready wrote in her journal that Morgan had stopped by on the previous evening, having been allowed no closer to Nashville than the asylum. There he and his men waited for an answer from a communication to General Buell and enjoyed the "elegant hospitality" of Mary Ready Cheatham, about whom he was "quite enthusiastic."[26]

In a speech given the day after his arrival in Nashville, Johnson stated that his purpose was to restore Tennessee to the Union through submission to the U.S. Constitution and laws; he offered amnesty to those swearing allegiance to the U.S. government. His policy was based on the premise, shared by Lincoln, Buell, and other Union commanders, that the great majority of Tennesseans were loyalists at heart, but had been forced into secession or misled by the duplicity of

---

[23] James Welch Patton, Unionism and Reconstruction in Tennessee, 1860-1868 (Chapel Hill: University of North Carolina Press, 1934), 30.
[24] Ibid., 31.
[25] Ibid., 22-23.
[26] C. Alice Ready, Diary, 49, Southern Historical Collection, University of North Carolina, Chapel Hill.

those in command. Johnson's plan for restoring Tennessee to the Union was twofold. He would silence the secessionist opposition by removing its leaders and by gaining control of the press; and he would encourage pro-Union sentiment by holding mass meetings of loyalists.[27]

Johnson moved swiftly, first appointing to his cabinet and staff Edward H. East, Secretary of State; Joseph S. Fowler, Comptroller; Horace Maynard, Attorney-General; and Edmund Cooper, private secretary and confidential agent.[28] He then required all office holders to take the loyalty oath long required by Tennessee's constitution. On March 27, the city council returned the oath forms unsigned. Two days later, Johnson ordered Colonel Stanley Matthews, the provost marshal, to arrest Mayor Cheatham.[29] Meanwhile, General Buell left with his army for Pittsburgh Landing and Secretary of State Edwin Stanton ordered General Halleck to secure Nashville.[30]

On March 30, Federal authorities began rounding up those who had publicly supported the Confederates. Most prominent were William G. Harding of Belle Meade, Judge Josephus Conn Guild of Sumner County, and Washington Barrow. All three, after refusing the oath, were sent North and imprisoned at Fort Mackinac, Michigan, for the summer. Using procedures established in 1861 by Confederates occupying Knoxville, Federals arrested a subject and offered parole which must be secured by $10,000. Although those refusing were under threat of death, they were usually either imprisoned locally, sent out of the state for the duration of the war, or sent to prison north of the Ohio River.[31]

On April 7, at the height of the battle of Shiloh or Pittsburgh Landing, Governor Johnson took over the government of Nashville, dismissing Mayor Cheatham, six aldermen, and fifteen councilmen. He retained three councilmen who had taken the oath, including William S. Cheatham, a cousin of the mayor. On April 10, he arrested five Protestant ministers and then released them on their own

---

[27] Patton, 34-35.
[28] Ibid., 34; Hall, 42.
[29] Durham, Nashville, 63-64; Graf, The Papers of Andrew Johnson, Vol. 5, 253.
[30] Durham, Nashville, 68.
[31] Graf, Papers, Vol. 5, xlvi; Durham, Nashville, 71-72.

recognizance. Johnson then turned his attention to the press, bringing unionist S. C. Mercer from Kentucky to publish the Daily Union. The first issue appeared on April 13. In the interim, he arrested and imprisoned the editors of the opposition press.[32]

During the week ending May 3, the provost guard arrested 2,000 secessionists, committing them to the state penitentiary or to a local jail.[33] Among them was Charles Ready, Jr., of Murfreesboro. Colonel John G. Parkhurst, commanding officer at Murfreesboro, wrote him a note on April 30, 1862, requiring him to take the oath. When Ready refused, he was taken to the penitentiary. Staying with the Ready family at the time was Mary Cheatham, whose sister Alice wrote "she is not very well and our time has all to be devoted to her."[34]

In mid-May, Johnson held mass meetings to stimulate unionist sentiment, but he suffered a major setback in his first test at the polls on May 22, when an anti-administration candidate, Turner S. Foster, won the post of circuit judge in the Nashville district. The invasion of cavalry detachments under Morgan and Forrest, combined with Johnson's own controversies with Buell, Halleck, and Rosecrans, postponed any further attempts at political reorganization of the state through elections.[35] Johnson returned, instead, to his program of bringing the secessionist leadership to heel.

Of all the groups, Johnson reserved his greatest ire for the secessionist clergy. On June 16, 1862, he ordered R. B. C. Howell, influential pastor of the First Baptist Church, two other ministers, and two physicians who may have been summoned by mistake, to appear in the office of Secretary of State Edward H. East. The two physicians were Dr. William A. Cheatham and Dr. W. B. Hall. East informed them that they had been called for the purpose of signing an oath of allegiance to the United States government. The ministers requested time to consider the matter, receiving twenty-four hours. Returning the next day with other ministers, but without the physicians, they demanded to see the governor. Andrew Johnson, who was highly excited, received

---

[32] Durham, Nashville, 73-76.
[33] Ibid., 148.
[34] C. Alice Ready, Diary, 90, 88.
[35] Patton, 36.

them. Dr. C. D. Elliott of the prestigious First Presbyterian Church presented their case. Afterwards Johnson

> turned upon them "with the fury of an enraged tiger, and told them they were all traitors, and that as to Mr. Elliott he ought to be hung. . . . He used the most violent and vituperative terms. . . . . The style, and spirit of the Governor, resembled very much those of an angry overseer, speaking to a herd of grossly offending slaves.[36]

On June 28 Howell and three other ministers reappeared in the Governor's office as ordered and refused to take the oath, whereupon they were taken to the penitentiary after again refusing the oath in the office of Lieutenant Colonel R. W. McClain, acting provost marshal. The others were sent to federal prison in the North, but Howell was so ill that he was sent home. His health and the prosperity of his church were virtually destroyed by the occupation.

East had told Howell that Johnson had devised a schedule for calling all the citizens of Nashville to take the oath. First were bankers and insurance men whom he had begun bringing in in April; second on the list were ministers; doctors, next; and so on through the entire population.[37]

If Cheatham and Hall had been erroneously called with the ministers, their turn would come soon. To make matters worse, an informant who identified himself only as "a Union man" sent the following letter to Andrew Johnson on June 26, 1862:

> [Nashville] June 26, 1862
>
> To Gov Johnson
> State of things at the insane asylum
>> this time last summer I heard doctor and Mrs Cheatham and old man ready say that King harris mist it by leting andy Johnson the treator go that he should be hung-- now sir them

---

[36] Rufus B. Spain, "R. B. C. Howell: Nashville Baptist Leader in the Civil War Period," <u>Tennessee Historical Quarterly</u> XIV (1955): 335. Dr. Elliott was also President of the Nashville Female Academy.
[37] Ibid.

very people are this very day I believe a stealing from the state[.] them have sent some three large chests to town one to cheathams wharehouse the other tow to Parrishes wharehoues[.] I am not certain what is in them but there are a grate many here that the[y] have just packed[.] I am told that tow contain ladys bolts of dry goods beding carpeting and so he has keep a bout, 3000. Pds. of rebel bacon that was stored here the time rebels run a way likewise 12 steers a large quantity of lard[.] you can find out if he has charged them to the state or not[.)   he keeps 12 hors here[.] the most of them is blood stock[.] he raisd the most of them here[.] he did get 2 carag horses from his brother in the rebel army[.] he did keep until lately a seamstress with 4 children to sew for his lady and the ready famaly[.] bill cheatham the gambler is out here[.] he was the first in nashville to raise a company the[y] caul the cheathe rifeles[.]   he stays out of the way here boarding at the docters No. 1 table[.] the famaly the[y] think the[y] are above all others[.] there is knothing is cared for here but the one table and the pachents can have knothing only the one thing all the time and I am told he dus not goe in to som of the wards in months[.] there is three cooking departments here one for the ladys the other for the gents the other for the superier negroes that cooks(.] the[y] can just dow as the[y please] in tow of them[.] I have not seen in four years the steward the docter or Mrs cheatham eather to order or see what the pachents got[.] the trustees dus not know anything about this[.] it is time that it was known to them and the public at large so as to make a change for the benefit of the poor inmates[.] the steward keeps the books[.] he is the man to keep until he lets the cat out of the bag[.] the docter has been one of the fourth or fifth on the rebel list in the gazette and ever since he has devoted all his time to help it[.]

from a Union Man[38]

---

[38] Graf, Papers, Vol. 5, 507-508. References in this letter are to the storage facilities of M.A. Parrish and Company, wholesale grocer; Dr. Cheatham's younger brother, Captain Boyd M. Cheatham; W. T. Cheatham of Marshall County, a first lieutenant

Dr. W. B. Hall, of the University of Nashville medical faculty, was arrested on June 10 and paroled to appear before the governor on June 21; he went into hiding in Kentucky. Thus he was unable to appear on June 30 when Dr. Elliott, Presbyterian minister and President of the Nashville Female Academy, Dr. J. P. Ford of the University of Nashville medical faculty, and Dr. William A. Cheatham, superintendent of the Tennessee Hospital for the Insane, were arrested, charged with treason, and committed to the penitentiary. Reportedly Cheatham's ill health earned him an immediate parole; however, this is more likely to have been the ill health of his wife. Doctors Elliott and Ford were sent to Camp Chase, Ohio.[39]

Morgan and Forrest kept Nashville virtually under siege during the summer of 1862. On July 13, Forrest received the surrender of Murfreesboro, and on July 22 he drew up his cavalry opposite the insane asylum, burning two railroad bridges and making prisoners of 83 prisoners nearby on Murfreesboro Pike.[40]

This action near the asylum may have reminded Andrew Johnson of a letter he had intended to write to Dr. Cheatham, as follows:

Nashville, July 25, 1862

Dr. Wm. A. Cheatham, Superintendent of the Tennessee Hospital for the Insane
>
> Dear Sir--The multiplicity of my duties have compelled me to delay giving that attention to the Tennessee Hospital for the Insane that its great importance demands. I hope, however, that no serious inconvenience has in consequence resulted to yourself. I am now happy to inform you that I am enabled to relieve you of your responsibility, and that you will pardon the delay.

---

in Cheatham's Rifles but not a close relative of Dr. Cheatham, and possibly not related at all; and Thomas Farmer from Springfield, who was the asylum steward.
[39] Durham, *Nashville*, 156.
[40] Ibid., 93.

> It is with pleasure that I am enabled to inform you, that Dr. W. P. Jones has been appointed to succeed you as Superintendent of the Hospital. You will be kind enough to deliver into his possession, the Institution, together with all the property of every kind connected therewith, which property belongs to the State.
>
> Respectfully, Andrew Johnson
> Military Governor [41]

Five days later, William B. Cassilly, acting provost marshal in Nashville, notified Johnson that he had seized "a very large quantity of boxes, containing clothing--bedding and furniture from the State Lunatic Asylum" which Dr. Cheatham had sent into town during the previous two days and asked for directions about what to do with it.[42]

On July 30, 1862, Mary Ready Cheatham wrote to her mother:

> I have left the asylum at last and I feel in my heart that I never wish to see the place again. No tongue can tell what I have suffered there within the last few months--and this last day was the climax of suffering. Mary told me this morning she was alarmed about me for the thought I would go crazy. Papa will tell you how we have been persecuted--I am very thankful my precious child [Martha Strong Cheatham] was with her dear Grand-ma and kind aunts. She will never know now [sic] of our troubles. Oh! I pray I may never have such trials again. Papa says he never knew before that I was so much like my mother. He tried lecturing me about controlling myself but for once in my life Papa's lectures were scarcely heeded by me. It was a comfort to have him with me, and Dr. C. was truly grateful that he was there. Just as soon as I can possibly get to you[,] Mama[,] I am going. Allie [her sister Alice] will stay with me until I can

---

[41] Graf, Papers, Vol. 5, 568
[42] Ibid.,568-569.

go. I cannot give her up to go with Papa. She has been <u>every</u> thing to me.[43]

Johnson may have been determined to destroy Dr. William A. Cheatham, but his destructive impulses did not extend to the institution itself. He selected a qualified physician as superintendent, Dr. William P. Jones. A prominent Unionist who was also a founder of Shelby Medical College, Nashville, Dr. Jones had taken charge of the Academy Hospital on March 1, 1862.[44] One of the Union fortifications, named "Fort Confiscation," was built around the residence of Dr. Jones. In December 1862, Union troops constructing the fort virtually destroyed his home, tore down the outbuildings, and removed the fences. They also cut down 20 acres of forest and 300 fruit trees and destroyed the shrubbery and gardens.[45]

Jones scarcely fared better at the asylum. In his report of 1865, he wrote movingly of his wartime trials. Two divisions of the Federal army had encamped on the asylum farm soon after his appointment. Despite orders to the contrary, the soldiers had burned the hospital's supply of wood and about five miles of cedar fencing. "Occasionally you might have seen, before daylight, the Superintendent, the farm hands, and a few patients, in the woods felling trees and hauling fuel to warm the house, that others might be comfortable," he wrote. Supplies were scanty, bills mounted, and a tornado lifted up a portion of the roof and blew it to the opposite side of the hospital. He, like Cheatham, complained of the hospital's location on a military thoroughfare, as well as the atmosphere of tension and unrest which led to staffing problems.[46]

On August 18, 1862, Governor Johnson distributed a circular assessing Confederate sympathizers sums ranging from $50 to $500

---

[43] Mary Ready Cheatham to Martha Strong Ready, 30 July 1862, Cheatham-Ready family papers in the possession of Mrs. H. Clinton Parrent and Mrs. Charles Bradley, Nashville.
[44] Durham, <u>Nashville</u>, 80.
[45] Ibid., 128-129.
[46] <u>Reports of the Trustees and Superintendent of the Tennessee Hospital for the Insane presented to the General Assembly, April 3, 1865</u> (Nashville: John T. S. Fall, 1865), 15-16.

payable in five days. The money would be used, he said, to pay the expenses of children and widows of misguided Tennesseans who had supported the Confederate cause. The list included the names of Archer and F. R. Cheatham, cousins of William A. Cheatham, each assessed $100; Mark R. Cockrill, assessed $200; and Byrd Douglas, the only man on the list assessed $500.[47]

Johnson expanded the concept and scope of his initial idea with an assessment for relief of the poor on December 13, 1862. The assessments were payable in five months, with the first payment due on or before December 20th. The first and largest assessment was of John Overton, for $2,500. William G. Harding, who had taken the oath and returned to Nashville in September, and Mark R. Cockrill were each assessed $1,000; J. A. S. Acklen and R. C. McNairy, $500; and Dr. W. K. Bowling, Dr. William A. Cheatham, and Archer Cheatham, $250 each. Johnson's aim was to levy a punitive tax on wealthy secessionists who had given money to the Confederacy. The list included eighty-four of Nashville's most affluent citizenry, several of whom had been refugees, and refugees were taxed in absentia.[48]

Nashville remained under siege throughout the fall of 1862. Confederate cavalry leader General Joe Wheeler kept telegraph lines down most of the time between August and November. Supplies in the city reached dangerously low levels. In early November, Generals Forrest and Morgan made a joint attack on the Nashville suburbs.[49] Although Rosecrans arrived in Nashville on November 11 to assume command of the Army of the Cumberland and supervise a buildup of Union troops, Confederate cavalry engaged Union forces in frequent skirmishes throughout November and December, culminating in Morgan's victory at Hartsville, Tennessee, on December 7.[50] Confederate morale was high in Middle Tennessee.

A rumor spread through the Army of Tennessee that Morgan intended to give the prisoners he had captured at Hartsville to 21-year-old Mattie Ready for a wedding present. The wedding, held at the Ready home in Murfreesboro on Sunday, December 14, was one of the great

---

[47] Graf, Papers, Vol. 5, 623-624.
[48] Ibid., Vol. 6, 97-99; Durham, Nashville, 164.
[49] Durham, Nashville, 117, 125-126.
[50] Ibid., 130-131, 134, 137.

social occasions of the Confederacy. Groomsmen were Mattie's brother, Horace Ready, an officer on General William J. Hardee's staff, and Col. George St. Leger Grenfell, an English soldier of fortune. General Leonidas Polk, who was an Episcopal bishop, performed the ceremony in his ecclesiastical robes while Generals Bragg, Hardee, Cheatham, and Breckinridge looked on with the headquarters staff. One of the two regimental bands playing outside came in to play for dancing after dinner. Meanwhile, Morgan's men, standing in front of the house on Main Street, built bonfires and cheered the newlyweds.[51]

President Jefferson Davis, in Murfreesboro the day before the wedding, had promoted Morgan to brigadier general. Eight days after the wedding, on December 22, General Morgan left on his famed Christmas raid, marching 500 miles in fourteen days and striking at the L&N line in a loop through Kentucky.[52] It was probably the apex of Morgan's career as a cavalry leader as well as the high point of the Confederacy in Middle Tennessee, where Morgan's wedding and the Christmas raid would always represent the romance and gallantry of the Lost Cause. But the Battle of Stone's River at Murfreesboro from December 31 to January 2, 1863, took the edge off Confederate hopes. Casualties poured into Nashville, Gallatin, and Murfreesboro; and Nashville alone contained twenty-five military hospitals.[53]

Rosecrans, who had established his winter headquarters in Nashville, supported Johnson's repression of Confederate sympathizers. He also introduced a new element when he introduced military secret police under Colonel William Truesdail in the late fall of 1862. Truesdail set up his office in the home of General Felix Zollicoffer at 28 High Street, where he became the most hated presence in the area.[54]

From the outset, Truesdail was a source of contention between Andrew Johnson and General Rosecrans. Among the charges leveled at Truesdail, who was a wealthy native of New York State living in Missouri before the war, was his practice of conducting personal

---

[51] James A. Ramage, Rebel Raider: The Life of General John Hunt Morgan (Lexington: University Press of Kentucky, 1986), 134.
[52] Ibid., 137.
[53] Durham, Nashville, 208.
[54] Ibid., 240.

business in army contracts. During the ten months he was in office, Truesdail ran a spy network that employed both male and female agents. One, A. B. Johnson, passed between Nashville and McMinnville, where General Morgan had established his headquarters. He delivered personal mail from Morgan's wife to her sister in Nashville, Mary Ready Cheatham. A. B. Johnson supplied Morgan with misleading information about the Federal army at Nashville. Morgan became suspicious of Johnson after his brother was arrested. In turn, Morgan arrested Johnson, but set him free when a court-martial failed to convict him. Truesdail then had Johnson arrested so that he could gather information from Confederate sympathizers in the penitentiary.[55]

The letter from Mattie Morgan to Mary Cheatham is a long one, affectionate, full of family news, and contains nothing of any military interest whatsoever. After the secret police copied the letter, Johnson delivered it to the Cheathams in the middle of the night. He agreed to return in a day or two to pick up letters and notions for Mrs. Morgan. These letters, too, were harmless.

Mary's letter to Mattie, dated February 20, 1863, told how the doorbell had rung at 2:30 a.m. to admit Johnson with the cherished letter. "I shall never get over not seeing you a bride," she wrote, still sad because she had not been able to attend the wedding in Murfreesboro. But she reminded her sister that she had fallen in love with Mattie's "dear, good husband" first, that day she had seen him on the turnpike in his blouse and coonskin cap. Mary was worried about her husband, who was in Louisville, where he had gone to bring back a slave named Penny to Mrs. Ready, his mother-in-law, in Murfreesboro.

Her letter was poignant testimony to the dismal state of affairs in Nashville:

> We don't see the bright side here, Mattie. It is nothing but gloom. When our prisoners come in we are sad, and go to work to clothe and feed them. These horrid prisons would make your heart sick. Hospitals on every street; and our poor wounded Confederates, how they did suffer! Many of them froze to death

---

[55] Ibid., 240-241.

at Camp Douglas [in Chicago]. . . . They were sent here on boats [in] that severe weather. Many of them were in a dying condition when they started. . . . Poor Mrs. McNairy has Frank's body in the house yet. It was embalmed. She is afraid to bury it.

She wrote, too, of the terrible disappointment after Stone's River. "Poor old Rutherford County! Such devastation! The people have been robbed of everything. Speaking of robbing, my horses have been taken," she added. "I never expect to have another pair, for when the war is over all the horses will be dead. I prized my horses very highly, and tried so hard to keep them."[56]

Federal authorities subjected Nashvillians to a wave of searches, seizures, and arrests during the first six months of 1863. Preceding large-scale arrests in April, 1863, was a rumor that authorities were on the verge of arresting 500 persons suspected of treason. As many as 125 citizens were under arrest by April 17, and during the week of May 5-13 Union officials sent many of the citizens to northern prisons.[57]

Among them were Dr. and Mrs. William A. Cheatham, whom Truesdail accused of passing information to General Morgan in February. On May 13, 1863, Nashville lawyer John S. Brien sent the following telegram to Governor Johnson, who was in Washington: "Dr. Cheatham and wife are ordered to Alton prison tomorrow morning(.] It is of the utmost importance to your plans here that he not be sent off until after your return[.] telegraph Gen Rosecrans at Murfreesboro to Suspend the order until you can get home--your presence here is very important[.]"[58]

Apparently the Cheathams' testimony would have aided Johnson in his campaign against Truesdail.[59] Union authorities sent the Cheathams to Louisville en route to prison in Alton, Illinois; but when Mrs. Cheatham became too ill to travel, they kept the Cheathams and their two children under house arrest at a hotel in Louisville. On May

---

[56] John Fitch, Annals of the Cumberland (Philadelphia: J. B. Lippincott & Co., 1864), 570-571.Fitch served as Provost Judge during the occupation.
[57] Durham, Nashville, 246-249.
[58] Graf, Papers, Vol. 6, 224.
[59] Ibid., 225.

18, Colonel Mundy, Post Commander, reported to Captain A. C. Semple, Assistant Adjutant General:

> I respectfully report that Dr. Cheatham, wife and children arrived this inst. on Saturday evening last in charge of an officer with orders to conduct them to Alton, Illinois, where they are to be confined in prison until the end of the war by order of Maj. General Rosecrans. No train leaves Louisville north on Sundays until 9 o'clock p.m. And I found Mrs. Cheatham who has been ill for some time unable to proceed further at present without great danger to her life. I sent the Medical Director Dr. Goldsmith to see her and I have not yet received his report today. I ordered the family to be left here in my custody until Mrs. Cheatham was able to be on the journey, which the officer in charge accordingly did, and the surgeon attending her has orders to report her as soon as she may be strong enough to bear the journey.[60]

On May 26, 1863, Andrew Johnson, who was by then in Louisville, telegraphed Col. Joseph Holt, Judge-Advocate-General, as follows: "Colonel Mundy, post commander here, has Doctor Cheatham and wife in custody until Mr[s]. Cheatham is able to travel. Please telegraph him an order to hold them here until further orders from the War Department or General Rosecrans."[61]

That same day, Edward R. S. Canby, Brigadier General and Assistant Adjutant-General at the War Department in Washington, telegraphed Major General W. S. Rosecrans, commanding the Department of the Cumberland, in Murfreesboro: "The Secretary of War has received your telegram of the 23rd instant and directs that you proceed with the execution of the sentence against Doctor and Mrs. Cheatham." He also telegraphed Colonel Mundy, Commanding at Louisville:

---

[60] National Archives, RG 109, War Department Collection of Confederate ·Records, Entry 465 (M345), "Cheatham, Dr. and Mrs."
[61] U. S. War Department, <u>The War of the Rebellion: A Compilation of the Official Records of the Union and Confederate Armies</u>, Series II, Vol. V, 709.

General Rosecrans reports that Doctor Cheatham and wife entertained a spy from General Morgan; sent letters and goods through lines and advised spy to dress in Federal uniform; go about city and learn and inform Morgan where our stores were located and where our troops were posted. General Rosecrans has been directed to proceed with the execution of this sentence. Please inform Governor Johnson.[62]

Meanwhile, also on May 26, 1863, M. Goldsmith, Surgeon and Superintendent of Hospitals, reported to the beleaguered Colonel Mundy:

I hereby certify that I have carefully examined Mrs. Dr. Cheatham, a prisoner, and find her in such a condition that in my opinion her removal would endanger her life, and that her confinement to a military prison, in her present condition of health, would be an act of simple inhumanity.[63]

On June 8, 1863, Colonel William Truesdail, Chief of Army Police, himself relented in a letter written from Murfreesboro to Colonel Goddard, Adjutant General:

Colonel:
 I have, during the several days past, been called upon by many friends and sympathizers of Dr. W. A. Cheatham & wife to solicit from the military authorities a change in the sentence of the Major General Commanding--from that of being sent to Alton Prison during the continuance of the present war--to that of a privilege of taking the Oath of Allegiance and of giving any Bond required for their loyalty and good behavior hereafter.
 In discovering and investigating the acts and conducts of Mr. & Mrs. Cheatham I was very careful to lay nothing before the General Commanding that I did not know to be positively true, in order that I should not be made responsible for doing

---

[62] Ibid.
[63] National Archives, RG 109, War Department Collection of Confederate Records, Entry 465 (M345), "Cheatham, Dr. and Mrs."

them any act of injustice, although, the while, both they and their friends, intimate and otherwise, have denounced me in terms of extreme bitterness.

Yet I am of the opinion that the relief now earnestly sought for, at your hands, may be mercifully extended without detriment to the Government.

> I am, Colonel
> Your Obt. Servt
> Wm Truesdail
> Chief Army Police[64]

As late as June 18th, military correspondence was still circulating in Louisville about the proper disposition of the Cheathams,[65] but as soon thereafter as Mrs. Cheatham was able to travel, they returned to Nashville.

In July, 1863, Nashvillians learned that Union cavalry had captured General John Hunt Morgan with most of his men in Ohio. Yet guerilla activity around Nashville remained strong during the summer and into the fall.[66] At the end of September, Nashville hospitals were overflowing with wounded from the Battle of Chickamauga. By the end of October, 4,800 refugees had passed through Nashville.[67] Grant's victory at Chattanooga on November 25 was a blow to Confederate sympathizers. But the dramatic escape of General Morgan with six of his men from Camp Chase, the military prison in Columbus, Ohio, improved their morale.

While in prison, Morgan corresponded frequently with his wife and her family, often mentioning the Cheathams, especially Mary. In mid-August, the Cheathams were in Nashville, but on August 30 Morgan had learned from his mother-in-law, Mrs. Ready, that Mary and the children were visiting in Murfreesboro. Mary's sister Ella had reported that Mary "met with a great many kind friends in Louisville,

---

[64] Ibid.
[65] Ibid.
[66] Walter T. Durham, <u>Reluctant Partners: Nashville and the Union, July 1, 1863, to June 30, 1865</u> (Nashville: Tennessee Historical Society, 1987), 2, 7.
[67] Ibid., 27, 29.

was quite ill but was entirely recovered".[68] On 13 September Morgan had learned that the Cheathams were well. Dr. Cheatham's brother, Foster, was "still in this place with us," Morgan commented wryly.[69]

On November 9, however, Morgan wrote Mrs. Ready in Murfreesboro, "I regret so much to hear that Mrs. Cheatham is still indisposed. She has had a sad time for several months. Should like so much to see her. Well remember the last time I had that pleasure and to her two sweet little ones give much love, and a kiss to each."[70] Although Mrs. Ready had reported that Mary was "very feeble," she was "much better than she has been,"[71] and her condition continued to improve, as evidenced by a letter Mary wrote to her brother-in-law Foster, which he received on November 18th.[72] Early in December Mattie learned from her brother-in-law, Charlton Morgan, who passed on news from a letter her mother had written to General Morgan, that Mrs. Ready had been in Nashville with Mary, who had been quite unwell.[73]

In late November, Grant established his headquarters in Nashville, where Federal officers and their families increasingly began using private homes as quarters. On December 3, General Lovell H. Rousseau, commander of the district of Nashville, complained to headquarters, Department of the Cumberland, that Federal officials

---

[68] John Hunt Morgan to Martha Ready Morgan, 30 August 1863, John Hunt Morgan Papers in the Southern Historical Collection, University of North Carolina, Chapel Hill.
[69] John Hunt Morgan to Martha Ready Morgan, 13 September 1863, John Hunt Morgan Papers in the Southern Historical Collection, University of North Carolina, Chapel Hill.
[70] John Hunt Morgan to Martha Strong Ready (Mrs. Charles Ready, Jr.), 9 November 1863, John Hunt Morgan Papers in the Southern Historical Collection, University of North Carolina, Chapel Hill.
[71] John Hunt Morgan to Martha Ready Morgan, 10 November 1863, John Hunt Morgan Papers in the Southern Historical Collection, University of North Carolina, Chapel Hill.
[72] John Hunt Morgan to Martha Ready Morgan, 18 November 1863, John Hunt Morgan Papers in the Southern Historical Collection, University of North Carolina, Chapel Hill.
[73] Charlton H. Morgan to Martha Ready Morgan, 7 December 1863, John Hunt Morgan Papers in the Southern Historical Collection, University of North Carolina, Chapel Hill.

were appropriating private dwellings and furniture and simply turning the owners out.[74]

The weather was bitter cold and fuel was scarce. In early December, Mrs. Ulysses S. Grant, who had joined her husband in Nashville, learned from her friend, Mrs. Peter M. Dix, that

> Dr. Cheatham, the most distinguished physician in the city and at the head of the insane asylum, whose wife had been confined to her bed for several years, had received an order from one of General Grant's staff officers, General William F. Smith, to vacate his house at once, as he wished it for himself and his wife. When I told General Grant he said, "Oh, no! There is some mistake. Smith would not do such a thing when he knows that I, a commanding officer, have taken two rooms only and am boarding with a family so as not to incommode anyone. He would hardly move anyone out of his home. You are misinformed; Smith is a gentleman and would not be guilty of such an act."
>
> When my friend called again, I told her what the General had said, but she replied, "There is no mistake. They are now preparing to move and are looking for quarters for themselves, and Mrs. Cheatham is very ill in consequence." I said, "Send the Doctor to see General Grant, and then he will believe." So Dr. Cheatham called and told General Grant, but the General could scarcely credit it even then, saying, "I cannot understand it. It is so unlike what I thought of Smith. Could there be any personal reason?" "No," Dr. Cheatham said, "unless it is because I happen to be the brother-in-law of John Morgan, who has been on a raid through Ohio and Indiana." The General gave him a safeguard which amply protected his home, and Smith went east soon afterwards.[75]

In late April a Nashville newspaper published the following obituary: "Died, on the morning of the 27th inst., Mary Ready, wife of

---

[74] Durham, Reluctant Partners, 41.
[75] John Y. Simon, ed., The Personal Memoirs of Julia Dent Grant (Mrs. Ulysses s. Grant) (New York: G. P. Putnam's Sons, 19 75), 127.

Dr. William A. Cheatham, of this city." The notice referred to her "extended circle of acquaintances," adding that her friends loved her for "those habits and traits of character which make even strangers feel as though with a tried and trusted friend." The notice concluded, "As a wife and mother, she was the pride and joy of her household, and her death has created a void in that once happy family which only time can efface."[76]

On May 22, her family sent a telegram to General Morgan in Augusta, Georgia, notifying him that "our dear sister Mary died in Nashville April 27th," and asking "where will letters reach you on matters?"[77] On August 14, Ella Ready wrote to her sisters Alice and Mattie:

> She died with rheumatism of the heart and had dreadful spells which were very painful, and almighty God forbid that I shall ever see another sister or brother suffer as she did for eight months. She talked to me a great deal about the brightness of the future for her, before anyone suspected that she thought she would soon leave us. Often in the stillness of the night she would have me to get the prayer book and we would have prayer together.
>
> She would often say that she would never get over not seeing Mattie a bride, but then she would brighten up and say, "but we will be happy when they all get home."
>
> Brother Will [Dr. Cheatham] has a very fine practice now and has his room at the office, and boards with Mrs. Washington, the children are with us and have grown so much that you will be perfectly astonished to see them, they are such darlings and comforters.[78]

---

[76] Ready family papers in the possession of Andrew c. Buddenhagen, Murfreesboro.
[77] Ready family telegram to General John Hunt Morgan in Augusta, Georgia, 22 May 1864, John Hunt Morgan Papers in the Southern Historical Collection, University of North Carolina, Chapel Hill.
[78] Ella L. Ready to "My darling Sisters" [Alice and Martha], 14 August (1864], John Hunt Morgan Papers in the Southern Historical Collection, University of North Carolina, Chapel Hill.

In a letter of February 19, 1865, Mrs. Ready wrote to Mattie Morgan in Augusta about the kindness of General Lovell H. Rousseau at the time of Mary's death: "it was through him alone that we were allowed the privilege of being with your beloved 'Sis' during her last moments: and a privilege indeed she considered it, for her faint voice was heard daily pronouncing blessings on his head." She reported that Dr. Cheatham came to see them frequently, "finds no place like home he says, but. . . I doubt if he ever finds another home as comfortable and sweet as the one he had, for although Mary was my daughter, I do not hesitate to say that she was a model wife and housekeeper, always thinking of her husband's comfort. The Dr. is very affectionate and perfectly devoted to the children." The letter, she concluded, was "General Rousseau's kindness, too, he told me he would send it, and to say what I pleased."[79]

Mary's death was only the first loss to strike the Ready family. On September 4, 1864, a private in the Union army shot and killed John Hunt Morgan in Greeneville, Tennessee.[80] On that same day, Atlanta fell. President Lincoln and Andrew Johnson proclaimed a day of prayer and Thanksgiving on September 11 to celebrate these two events, as well

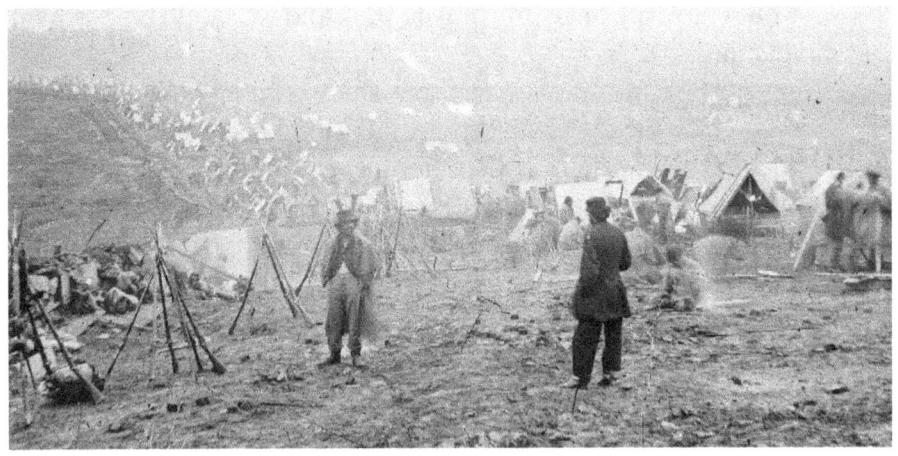

Battle of Nashville, Union Lines. Courtesy of the Library of Congress.

---

[79] Martha Strong Ready to Martha Ready Morgan, 19 February 1865, John Hunt Morgan Papers in the Department of Library Special Collections, Manuscripts, Western Kentucky University, Bowling Green.
[80] Ramage, 237.

as Wheeler's retreat from Nashville; but to those on the Confederate side it was a day of mourning.

Events quickly moved towards the inevitable conclusion. In November 1864, Lincoln won a second term in the presidency with Andrew Johnson elected as his vice-president. The Confederate army made its final retreat from Middle Tennessee after the Battle of Nashville on December 15 and 16, 1864. In early March 1865, those Tennesseans who qualified to vote elected Brownlow governor of Tennessee, while Andrew Johnson took the oath as vice-president of the United States. Lee surrendered on April 9, Lincoln was assassinated on April 15, and on May 29 President Johnson issued a proclamation of pardon and amnesty which "led progressively to his proclamation of unconditional pardon and amnesty in 1868."[81]

In retrospect, the program of Andrew Johnson and President Lincoln achieved the results they had hoped for in Tennessee. They had significantly altered both the leadership and institutions of the state, restoring it to the Union through elections without ever subjecting it to the harsh effects of Radical Reconstruction. That Middle Tennessee society had suffered a severe disruption is clearly evident in the lives of Dr. William A. Cheatham and his family.

Mary Ready Cheatham and her brother-in-law, John Hunt Morgan, are examples of the most severe loss, that of life itself, on both the civilian and military level. Mary's loss was private, deeply felt by her husband, two young children, and a wide circle of friends. The Confederacy at large mourned the death of Morgan, whose daring raids kept hope alive when significant defeats were occurring on major battlefields.

Dr. Cheatham is an example of the disruption of career and loss of position that afflicted many southern men during the war. He had moved the first patients into the new Tennessee Hospital for the Insane in 1852, and had devoted ten of his most productive years to the creation of a leading institution in his region and the country. He was beginning to develop a national reputation in the new field which would later be called psychiatry, when the war dashed his ambitions and returned him, permanently, to private practice.

---

[81] Durham, Reluctant Partners, 301.

Like Cheatham, the institution which he represented fell on hard times after the war. This was partially the result of a lack of funds, but it was also a result of disturbed momentum. Medical developments in neurology and a new attitude of pessimism resulting from the war led to a decreased confidence in the theory of moral treatment practiced by Cheatham and his colleagues. By 1870 virtually all institutions for the mentally ill had become custodial. The era of optimism was over.

For others, there was a general narrowing of options. Colonel Horace Ready, Mary's brother, and General B. F. Cheatham, Dr. Cheatham's cousin, were military men out of work and looking for new careers in a state that offered little economic opportunity.

Despite the devastating effects of the war on their private and professional lives, this family persisted by adapting to new circumstances. Dr. Cheatham established a private practice which he continued almost to the year of his death, in 1900. In 1867 he remarried, choosing as a wife the wealthy Adelicia Acklen, mistress of Belmont, reclaiming at least a home and an affectionate mother for his children. He saw his daughter married to Thomas Weaver and his son educated at the University of Virginia and Bellevue Hospital in New York; he lived to enjoy his grandchildren. But he never regained the public and professional standing he had enjoyed as superintendent and physician of the Tennessee Hospital for the Insane.

Mattie Morgan remarried, raised the daughter she had borne to Morgan, and represented her husband as the widow of a Lost Cause hero. Mattie died in 1887, at the age of 46; her daughter, Johnnie, died a year later, leaving no direct descendants of John Hunt Morgan.[82]

Colonel Horace Ready is an example of the versatility which desperate circumstances brought out in so many southerners. Deprived of the traditional slave labor supply, he signed a sharecropper contract with a freedman. Cash was so short that both agreed to split the cost of shoeing the mule that would draw the plow. Eventually Horace Ready turned the family home into a boarding house, keeping a ledger of those who came to dinner and to spend the night.[83]

---

[82] Ramage, 255.
[83] Ready family papers in the possession of Andrew C. Buddenhagen, Murfreesboro.

General B. F. Cheatham served through the entire war without injury. When it was over, he married Elizabeth Robertson and successfully ran a stock farm which his father-in-law gave them at Noah, midway between Beech Grove and Manchester. Cheatham ran for office, but was defeated. He received two appointments, one to the postal service and another as superintendent of the penitentiary. Perhaps he was the most successful at adapting to post-war life. But he never quite regained his former prosperity, status, or power. His son, also a general named Benjamin Franklin Cheatham, was reintegrated into the tide of national affairs, but with distinctly southern overtones. Following his military career he became superintendent of General Lee's home, Stratford, and a custodian of the Lost Cause.

Stephen Ash sees the Middle Tennessee experience as "passage from the old world to the new."[84] Furthermore, he views the passage as a regressive step for the white population, which became "more rural, more agrarian, more hidebound than it had been a decade earlier."[85] Ash's study of Middle Tennessee leads him to conclude that "the genesis of the progressive, bourgeois New South lies elsewhere than in the Civil War and Reconstruction."[86] A study of the Cheatham and Ready family members bears this out: their story is one of attempting to cope with, and accommodate to, a major upheaval that destroyed much of the momentum in their lives and forced them into unforeseen roles.

Other historians share Ash's view. J. G. Randall and David Donald, in The Civil War and Reconstruction, wrote that "the South had been broken by the war."[87] They cite an English traveler, Robert Somers, who wrote that "many who were once the richest among their fellows have disappeared from the scene, and few have yet risen to take their place."[88] A quarter of a million soldiers had died, as well as a large number of civilians "who perished as a by-product" of the war. "What

---

[84] Ash, 251.
[85] Ibid., 252.
[86] Ibid.
[87] James G. Randall and David Donald, The Civil War and Reconstruction, 2d ed. (Boston: D. c. Heath & Co., 1961), 543.
[88] Ibid., 544.

had taken place was the collapse of a civilization," they state unequivocally.[89]

"For most Southerners, Lee's surrender did not mark the end of life but the beginning of a difficult period of readjustment to new conditions,"[90] Randall and Donald point out. Like members of the Cheatham and Ready families, other southerners began rebuilding what had been lost. "Promising as this rehabilitation was, it did not keep up with the phenomenal industrial progress of the rest of the country," so that the South remained essentially an agricultural region with a new system of labor, sharecropping.[91] This was hardly progress; it was disruption on a major scale, although there were, of course, exceptions.[92]

The psychological effects of defeat and, for Middle Tennessee experiencing an "early Reconstruction," the trauma of occupation, are incalculable. Inevitably they must have produced an instinct to withdraw, much as an injured animal slinks off to lick its wounds. Despite such traumatic factors as loss of life, destruction of career, and narrowing of options, Dr. Cheatham and his extended family demonstrated essential vitality and underlying strength in the ways they adapted to new circumstances. But clearly they suffered a setback of major proportions. The war wrenched them "out of one historical epoch and into another"[93] during a period of only a few years and forced them to come to terms with a new way of life.

---

[89] Ibid., 545.
[90] Ibid., 547.
[91] Ibid., 548, 550.
[92] One of the most striking was the Nashville widow, Adelicia Hayes Franklin Acklen, who managed, with the help of her cousin, Sarah A. Gaut, and the aid of both Union and Confederate authorities, to export 2,000 bales of cotton from her seven Louisiana plantations to England in 1864. There it sold for $2,000,000. Albert W. Wardin, Jr., Belmont Mansion, The Home of Joseph and Adelicia Acklen (Nashville: Historic Belmont Association, 1981), 21-22.
[93] Gavin Wright, The Political Economy of the Cotton South (1978), quoted in C. Vann Woodward, Thinking Back: The Perils of Writing History (Baton Rouge: Louisiana State University Press, 1986), 77.

CHAPTER 6
WHEN THE WAR WAS OVER:
DR. CHEATHAM AND ADELICIA ACKLEN DURING RECONSTRUCTION AND THE GILDED AGE

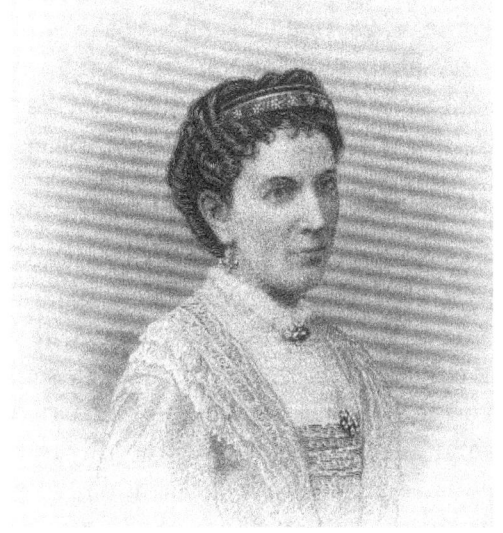

Mrs. Adelicia Cheatham. From *Queens of American Society* published in 1867.

On a June evening in 1867, a brilliant reception took place in Nashville, Tennessee, at the estate called Belle Monte. The hosts had invited 1,500 guests to the elaborate affair, which reputedly cost $10,000, an amazing sum to spend on a social event in a state yet to emerge from Reconstruction. The reception celebrated the marriage on June 18, 1867, of Belle Monte's owner, Adelicia Hayes Franklin Acklen, one of the wealthiest women in the state and in the South, to William Archer Cheatham, a physician from one of the oldest and most well established Tennessee families.

    No matter that the bride was fifty years old, the same age her first bridegroom, Isaac Franklin, the slave trader, had been when she married him in 1839. She was richly dressed in a gown of heavy white silk, with a veil of Brussels point lace flowing over her shoulders, a coronet given to her by the Emperor and Empress of France resting on her head, and a diamond clasp fastening the girdle encircling her waist.[1] One guest, when asked if the dark-haired Adelicia had retained her beauty, replied, "It could not be seen for the flash of gems--neck, brow, arms, hands and waist were blinding with the glitter of diamonds."[2]

The bridegroom standing at her side in the receiving line was dressed starkly, by contrast, in a black suit accentuated only by a white waistcoat and tie. Three years younger than his bride, this widower with two children was very likely still the handsome man he had been in earlier years. But just as he stood in the shadow of Adelicia's opulent beauty at their wedding reception, so would he through the years of their marriage, which ended in a reportedly amicable separation within two years of her death in 1887.

Today William Archer Cheatham is known, if he is remembered at all, as the third and least significant of Adelicia Acklen's three husbands. The saying is that the first, slave trader and planter Isaac Franklin, she married for money; the second, Joseph Acklen, she married for love; and the third, Cheatham, she married for position.[3] To some it may seem unlikely that a woman recently returned from the court of France would need to enhance her position; but in actuality her European triumphs would have mattered little to Nashville society, where she needed a worthy consort. The one she chose was not only descended from the prominent Cheatham and Washington families of Robertson County, but he was also well educated, refined, and a perfect gentleman.

Dr. Cheatham was by no means a nonentity, however. Eclipsed by the dazzling Adelicia during the years of their marriage and in posterity, he was in some very important ways the most significant of Adelicia's husbands, though not in relation to her. He made a remarkable contribution, both as a physician pioneering in the new fields of psychiatry and mental health, and as superintendent of the Tennessee Hospital for the Insane, one of the major social reforms accomplished by the state government in the years immediately preceding the Civil War. These accomplishments, when viewed from

---

[1] Copy of 1867 Nashville newspaper clipping in possession of Dr. Mack Wayne Craig.
[2] <u>Nashville American</u>, 15 August 1909.
[3] Telephone interview with Irene Jackson Wills, 6 April 1988. Mrs. Wills is directly descended from Dr. William A. Cheatham.

the larger perspective of public service, overshadow those of Isaac Franklin and Joseph Acklen, both of whom committed their lives to making money and building large estates for themselves and their heirs.

Widowed during the war, Adelicia Acklen left for Europe soon after the surrender at Appomattox, taking her four children with her. While absent from Belle Monte, she often thought of home, and dreamed one night that she was in her greenhouse there. Despite the sights she had seen, she thought America "the most beautiful country after all." While in Europe, she bought additional works of art for Belle Monte. Returning to Nashville late in the year 1866, she resumed her social life, giving an opulent reception for her house guest, Madame Octavia Le Vert, on December 18.[4]

In the spring of 1867 it became known that she and Dr. William A. Cheatham were planning to marry.[5] One can only speculate about the circumstances of their courtship, which may have begun before Adelicia departed for Europe, or may have been only a few months or weeks in duration. Certainly they shared a strong mutual interest in horticulture, greenhouses, and fine paintings and sculpture. Both had children in their households; and while he does not appear to have left a noticeable impression on hers, his daughter, Martha Strong Cheatham, later admonished her grandchildren, "Don't believe stories about wicked stepmothers--I had a wonderful stepmother."[6]

The wedding took place at 8 p.m. on June 18, 1867, at Belle Monte;[7] the Reverend R. F. Bunting performed the ceremony. The day before, Adelicia and William A. Cheatham had signed a pre-nuptial contract conveying all of her property in trust to George W. Shields, who was married to her sister, Laura Hayes. In addition to Belle Monte, the property included a house and lot on Cherry Street in Nashville; a 1,250 acre plantation in Sumner County known as Fairview, which had belonged to her first husband, Isaac Franklin; six

---

[4] Eleanor Graham, "Belmont: 1. Nashville Home of Adelicia Acklen," <u>Tennessee Historical Quarterly</u> Vol. XXX, No. 4 (Winter 1971), 361-362.
[5] Ibid., 363.
[6] Interview with Mrs. Mary w. Parrent and Mrs. Martha w. Bradley, 27 April 1988.
[7] William B. Lawrence diary, 10 August 1867. "On June 18th at 8 a-clock Sister Ade was married to Dr. Cheatham."

plantations in West Feliciana Parish, Louisiana; two city lots in New York; and a vast amount of jewelry, plate, furniture, and paintings. Although Shields was trustee, the contract reserved for Adelicia the right, at any time during her marriage, to sell and convey any of the property, and to invest and re-invest it. She could also change the trustee at will. Because Tennessee law stipulated that a woman's property became her husband's at the time of marriage, Adelicia had used a similar pre-nuptial contract at the time of her marriage to Joseph Acklen, in order to avoid losing control of the estate she had inherited from Isaac Franklin; and she again used the device in order to retain control of her property when she married Cheatham. In the contract, Cheatham renounced his right to any community interest in her property, then or in the future, regardless of the laws of the various states.[8]

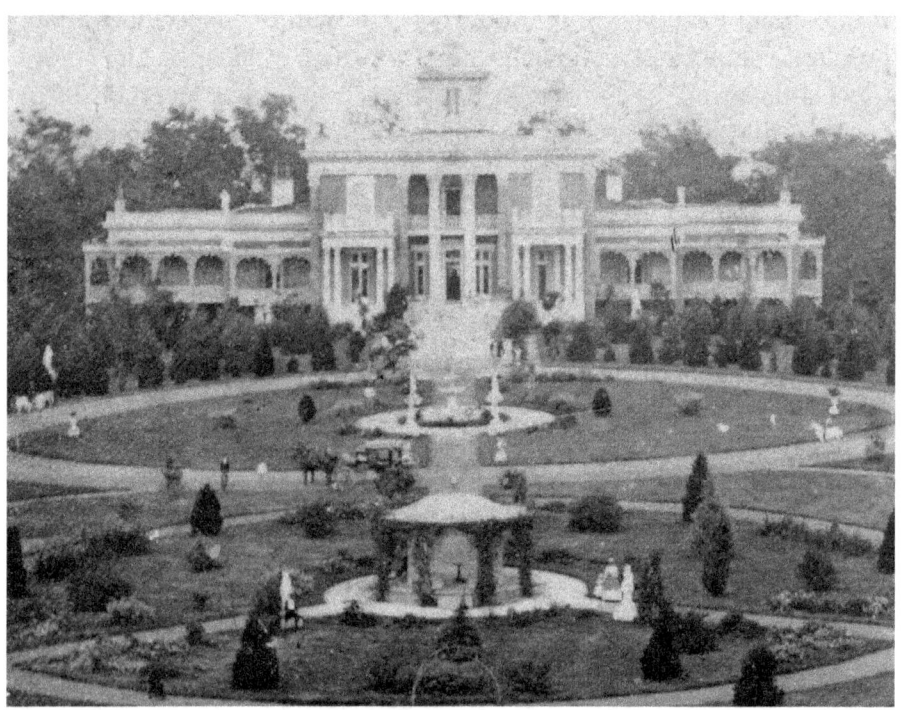

Belmont Mansion. Taken in 1865 by Morse & Peaslee, Gallery of the Cumberland. From the collection of the Belmont Mansion Association.

---

[8] Davidson County, Tennessee, Deed Book 38, 287.

The marriage began auspiciously. Adelicia ordered engraved calling cards and note cards with the monogram A and W interwoven over a C, encircled by a laurel wreath. Adelicia exerted herself in attempting to fill the role of mother to Cheatham's daughter, who was called Mattie. She wrote to her care of Colonel Ready, her grandfather, in Murfreesboro on July 31st, 1867, just over a month after the wedding: "My warm affection for your dear father would cause me to love his children but yours, and your brother's sweet loving dispositions but make it the more secure." Adelicia's Willie and the two little ones [Pauline and Claude] were at home. Dr. Cheatham and Mr. Shields had gone to Fairview the day before and were gone all day, "a very long one to me without him," she continued. They had taken evening drives and sometimes a visit in the country. Willie had the little buggy ready, had missed Richard, "and I think regretted not having gone with him" to Murfreesboro.[9]

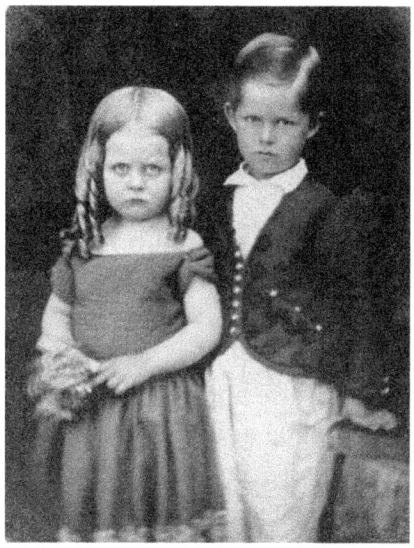 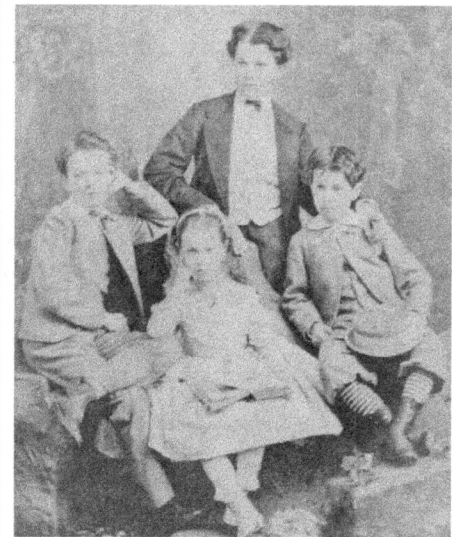

Left – Mattie and Richard Cheatham. Courtesy of a private collection.
Right – Joseph, William, Claude, and Pauline Acklen. 1865-66. From the collection of the Belmont Mansion Association.

---

[9] Adelicia Acklen to Martha Strong Cheatham, 31 July 1867, Cheatham-Ready family papers in the possession of Mrs. H. Clinton Parrent and Mrs. Charles Bradley, Nashville. Adelicia's four children were Joseph (b. 1850), William Hayes (b. 1855), Claude (b. 1857), and Pauline Acklen (b. 1859).

On Sunday, October 18, 1868, Adelicia wrote to Mattie at Patapsco Institute in Maryland. "My dear Child," she began, reporting that General and Mrs. Frank (B. F.) Cheatham had spent several days with them. She explained that General Cheatham, a cousin of her husband, had "decided to live at 'Fairview' which would relieve your Papa of the care as well as trips during the winter--and then it would be very pleasant for us to go up there next summer and spend several days at a time with them." Adelicia had been to church, but her husband had planned to go out to Mark Cockrill's with General Frank Cheatham. She had not written about Richard Cheatham's accident while out hunting. He and Willie Lawrence, one of Adelicia's nephews, had been out hunting, and the gun went off, wounding Richard in the shoulder. Dr. Cheatham had removed some of the shot from his son's shoulder, and Richard was nearly well as she wrote.

Adelicia added on Tuesday, October 19th, that she and Dr. Cheatham expected to go direct to New Orleans, then up to the plantation where they would remain a few days, and then go up the river to Memphis to attend Mollie Church's wedding which would take place the 18th next month. The mockingbird had died--he was dear to her because of associations, she wrote significantly.[10]

Adelicia's letter dated November 22, 1868, contained news of the wedding, a fire at Belle Monte, and news about domestic arrangements:

> We are now fixed for the winter in the little nursery. Pauline and Claude occupy one bed. It is very snug and comfortable, much more so than our large bedroom. Richie and Willie occupy the adjoining room--Joseph upstairs. We all congregate as usual in the little study at night or some of us in the nursery. I generally hear Claude and Pauline's lessons at night. They are progressing well.

She and Dr. Cheatham were planning to leave for Louisiana on the 5th of December in order to make necessary improvements on the

---

[10] Ibid., 18 October 1868.

plantation for another year. Mattie's Uncle Dick [Richard Cheatham, who had been mayor of Nashville when Union troops first occupied the city] and General Cheatham had been out that evening to Belle Monte. They had gone to the greenhouses and found a few camellias blooming.

Then Adelicia's letter to Mattie shifted to a more serious topic: "I will make Willie and Claude write. It has troubled your Papa and I-- this estrangement between you and Willie, and it must be remedied by mutual confidence. Claude has always loved you very much. You must all love one another my dear child, there is nothing more beautiful than family harmony and affection." Adelicia signed the letter, "Your Affectionate Mother."[11]

The following spring, on April 19th, 1869, William A. Cheatham began a letter "My precious child," reporting to Mattie that he had left Louisiana on March 31st, having found everything "getting along as well as could be expected on the plantations." He spoke of the beauty of Louisiana, where roses and spring flowers of every description were in bloom, while alligators sunned themselves in the bayous. He had spent two days in New Orleans where the state fair and races were going on. "You would enjoy being there at your age with your young feelings so fresh," he wrote, expressing the hope that Mattie could accompany them there every winter once her school days were over. "I miss you my darling child so much that it will be a happy day when I can again have you with us here at our happy and beautiful home," he concluded.[12]

Joseph Acklen had very actively managed Adelicia's properties, spending six to eight months a year on the Louisiana plantations.[13] She had begun her marriage with Cheatham by giving him the same kind of responsibility, culminating in her petition to the Davidson County Chancery Court with her husband, on April 19, 1870, in which she requested the resignation of George W. Shields, trustee, in favor of William A. Cheatham. The petition alleged that "since her intermarriage with the said William A. Cheatham that he has attended

---

[11] Ibid., 22 November 1868.
[12] Ibid., Dr. William A. Cheatham to Martha Strong Cheatham, 19 April 1869.
[13] Albert W. Wardin, Jr., Belmont Mansion, The Home of Joseph and Adelicia Acklen (Nashville: Historic Belmont Association, 1981), 8.

to her large business and property in the States of Tennessee, Louisiana and New York and elsewhere up to this time."[14]

Cheatham was accepted as trustee and ordered to report to the court on the 10th of October of each year regarding his actions; he was also ordered to submit his expenses to the court for compensation. During the October term of court, 1871, he duly submitted a lengthy report on the estate, stating that he had visited the Louisiana plantations in November, January, and April, where he had made contracts with the blacks for the upcoming cotton season. He used the proceeds of the last crop to stock Fairview and the Louisiana plantations, to make additional payments on the Tennessee Manufacturing Company's stock, and to pay taxes and general family expenses. He reported that the Fairview property was in good condition and "by judicious improvements increased in value, also the New York real estate in good paying condition and renting for five hundred dollars more per annum. He added that the Belle Monte place had undergone "material but necessary improvements" and was otherwise "almost self-sustaining." He appended to the report a five-year contract with Cleveland Scott for the management of the Fairview estate in Sumner County. There followed also an itemized list of expenses and credits related to the estate.[15]

A little over two months later, on the 23rd of December, 1871, Dr. and Mrs. Cheatham appeared before the Hon. E. H. East, Chancellor, to receive the report of the Clerk & Master relative to the amount of compensation due Dr. Cheatham for his year's work of managing the estate. After examining Dr. Cheatham's report as well as the deposition of Mr. George W. Shields, the brother-in-law of Adelicia who had previously served as trustee, the Clerk & Master concluded that Dr. Cheatham should be compensated in the amount of $2,500 for his services. This amount was considerably less than the $4,000 per annum previously paid to Mr. Shields. The Clerk & Master stated that the estate was being handled as it had been in previous years, and that Dr. Cheatham had discharged his duties "in a prudent and judicious manner. But he noted that Dr. Cheatham had paid his own expenses

---

[14] Davidson County, Tennessee, Chancery Court Minute Book Q, 468-470.
[15] Davidson County, Tennessee, Chancery Court Minute Book U, 52-53, 360-316.

out of the trust estate and that he was also paying $600 out of the trust estate for the services of a bookkeeper, whereas the former trustee had kept the books himself and paid his own family expenses. Thus Dr. Cheatham was awarded $2,500; he was also required to pay costs.[16]

On April 1, 1872, the new arrangement came to an abrupt end, when William A. Cheatham and wife again petitioned the court to accept the resignation of William A. Cheatham as trustee and reappoint George W. Shields. No explanation was offered and none was required by the court in granting the petition.[17] Almost anything could have happened to bring an end to Cheatham's participation in the management of Adelicia's estate. He could have tried to take more control than she was willing to give, or spent too lavishly, or been granted what she considered an excessive compensation. He could have tired of her excessive instructions, found the work too demanding and the travel too arduous, or the compensation insufficient; or he could simply have preferred to return to his medical practice. Whatever the reasons, they were kept private. Quite obviously Dr. Cheatham's duties in regard to Adelicia's property and her rigorous social schedule, involving numerous trips, would have made it virtually impossible for him to maintain the practice of medicine as long as he was trustee of Adelicia's property. But this impediment was removed in April of 1872 when Shields resumed his former post as trustee.

Mattie did eventually go to New Orleans, where she boarded and studied with Madame L. E. Cenas. On March 25, 1871, her stepbrother Claude had written her an affectionate note; the same envelope contained one from Adelicia, explaining that Pauline had posted one to her yesterday. Her father was in town--"fat and well," Adelicia wrote. Another letter dated March 25th was to Mattie from Willie. It was cordial but affected, and he probably wrote it under Adelicia's watchful eye.[18]

---

[16] Ibid. Chancellor East had been Andrew Johnson's Secretary of State during his military governorship of Tennessee (1862-18 65).
[17] Ibid., Book V, 90.
[18] Claude Acklen, Adelicia Acklen, and William Hayes Acklen to Martha Strong Cheatham, 25 March 1871, Cheatham-Ready family papers in possession of Mrs. H. Clinton Parrent and Mrs. Charles Bradley.

The letters Mattie so carefully saved give the picture of a harmonious family with parents who closely involved themselves in the lives of their children and who were themselves affectionate.

The only hint of discontent was the animosity between Willie and Mattie. The descendants of Dr. Cheatham uniformly report that the separation between the doctor and Adelicia, when Adelicia moved to Washington, D.C., with Pauline in 1885, was amicable. But one family member repeats a rumor that they had quarreled because Dr. Cheatham did not approve of the way Adelicia was bringing up her children.[19] A reading of the 458- page autobiography of William Hayes Ackland (Willie pretentiously changed his last name to the earlier English spelling of "Ackland") clearly reveals that Dr. Cheatham would have been on the right track in Willie's case, if indeed Dr. Cheatham made the criticism. From early childhood Willie was an over-indulged tyrant, the prototype of the spoiled rich brat. As an adult he was a professional socialite and international name-dropper. Nowhere in the entire manuscript does he mention his stepfather, Dr. Cheatham, or his stepbrother Richard, who was his age and with whom he was raised.[20]

Willie's animosity towards his stepsister and his need to be the center of his mother's attention did not prevent Mattie Cheatham from forming a close and affectionate relationship with her stepmother. In the spring of 1872 her father had relinquished control of his wife's affairs while he returned to the practice of medicine, which probably led to a divergence of interests as his wife pursued an active social life and travel schedule. Nonetheless, Adelicia hosted the wedding of Mattie Strong Cheatham to a young lawyer, Thomas S. Weaver, at Belle Monte on May 21 of 1872. The ceremony was performed at 12 noon by the Reverend Dr. Van Dyke, pastor of First Presbyterian Church, with relatives and nearest neighbors to witness the ceremony. After a lavish luncheon, the bride and groom left on an afternoon train for New York.[21] Mattie's brother, Richard, 17, would soon be attending the

---

[19] Interview with Mrs. David Y. Proctor, Nashville, Tennessee.
[20] William Hayes Ackland Autobiography, Manuscript #3547, in the Southern Historical Collection, University of North Carolina Library, Chapel Hill.
[21] Nashville Union and American, 22 May 1872, 4.

University of Virginia and then Bellevue Medical College in New York City, returning in 1877 to practice with his father.[22]

When Nashville celebrated its centennial in 1880, Dr. and Mrs. Cheatham both served on committees, she loaned paintings from Belmont, and he was officer on duty at the horticultural exhibit. They continued their round of entertainments, sponsorships, and trips into the fall. On October 4 Adelicia wrote her son William disconsolately that she "sits alone at the table," elaborating that at dinner she and Dr. Cheatham were the only people "in this big house." At the end of the year Adelicia and son William sold the rest of Angola to Samuel L. James, who held the lease for convict labor from the state of Louisiana and had been using that labor to farm her plantations. He and his partner, Louis Trager, paid $100,000, of which William received one-third; Adelicia assigned equal shares to Claude and Pauline in her will.[23]

While the Cheathams and Pauline were in New Orleans for Mardi Gras, her son Claude leased Fairvue to a Mr. Dunn without his mother's permission. In March she retained Thomas Weaver, Mattie's husband, to represent her in court to break the lease. After William left Belmont in June, Adelicia wrote to her son "it has turned cool, and Dr. Cheatham is reading his papers," conveying a degree of separation from her intellectual husband. In July, Dr. and Mrs. Cheatham, Joseph, Pauline, and Richard attended a ball in Monteagle where Adelicia, still glamorous at 64, shone in black satin d'Lyon brocade with diamonds. Later in the year the Cheathams traveled to Saratoga and New York City.[24]

February of 1882 found Adelicia and Pauline in New Orleans for Mardi Gras. Later in the spring it was announced that Dr. Cheatham would be resident physician for the summer at Bon Aqua, a new resort west of Nashville opening in June. Adelicia served on the invitation committee for the Grand Dress Ball at Bon Aqua on August 11th. In November she divested herself of Fairview, the home she had shared

---

[22] Brown, Mark et al. *Adelicia Acklen's Life in Chronological Order*. Unpublished manuscript Belmont Mansion research files, 2018, 1877/03/01. Richard was not licensed until 1889, the year before his father died.
[23] Warden, 31
[24] Brown, 1881/03/01, 1881/03/29, 1881/06/23, 1881/08/04

with Isaac Franklin, selling it to Charles Reed, a New Yorker who made his fortune as a blockade runner for the Confederacy.[25]

In 1883 Adelicia and Pauline attended Mardi Gras, followed by a trip to Florida accompanied by Dr. Cheatham.[26] In June, after Richard Cheatham married Emma Berry at her home on Franklin Pike, Dr. Cheatham returned to Bon Aqua for the summer.[27] Adelicia began work on a mausoleum at Mt. Olivet. In September she had the bodies of Isaac Franklin and their three younger children moved from Fairview to Mt. Olivet and placed temporarily in the Nelson vault. In November a committee visited Belmont to see if it would be suitable for a permanent exposition site—possibly a sign that Belmont, too, was for sale.[28] Change was in the air.

Because of the extremely cold weather in January 1884 the Cheathams and Pauline established their residence at the Maxwell House.[29] Dr. Cheatham continued to practice medicine with his son Richard at 16 South Cherry Street. Adelicia made out her will just before her 67th birthday on March 15th. Then she, Dr. Cheatham, and Pauline spent three weeks at the Ebbitt House hotel in Washington, D. C., where it was announced that Pauline had received much attention in Washington society.[30] After visiting Philadelphia and other eastern cities, all returned to the Maxwell House. Adelicia was a chaperone at the charity ball for the Working Women's Exchange at the Maxwell House, and her husband served on the gentlemen's reception committee.[31] On May 20th Pauline gave an evening tea for 20 guests at Belmont; the house was decorated with flowers within, "while from the lawn without floated the odor of new mown hay."[32]

In June Dr. Cheatham returned to Bon Aqua, where Adelicia and Claude visited at the end of July. In September it was announced

---

[25] Reid Smith, Majestic Middle Tennessee (Prattville, AL: Paddle Wheel Publications, c. 1975, reprint 1982): 133.
[26] Times- Picayune 2/18/1883
[27] Daily American 6/29/1883; Nashville Banner 6/29/1883
[28] Daily American 11/26/1883.
[29] Ibid., 11 January 1884.
[30] Ibid., 29 February 1884.
[31] Ibid., 23 April 1884.
[32] Ibid., *22 April 1884*

that the mausoleum at Mt. Olivet was to be completed at a cost of $11,000, and by the next spring Franklin and all four of their children had been placed in it. Both Cheathams attended a round of fall receptions, including one to assist their longtime friend Mrs. James K. Polk, and the third annual charity ball for the Working Women's Exchange. Then Adelicia, Pauline, William, and Claude left Nashville for Orlando to spend the winter. It was three days before Christmas.[33]

In April of 1885 Adelicia wrote that she had purchased some lots in Orlando. On May 31st it was reported that Dr. Cheatham, Adelicia, and Pauline had been visiting Washington and had taken a home on Iowa Circle. It was the last known time the Cheathams traveled together. July 27th was the last known time Adelicia was at Belmont, or in Nashville.[34]

Cheatham's residence continued to listed "in the country," that is to say Belmont, in the Nashville City Directory through 1885. In 1874 he had been listed as a partner in Liddard & Company, which dealt in drugs and medicine, and he continued to practice medicine with his son Richard at 16 South Cherry Street. A few years earlier, in May of 1881, Dr. Cheatham showed a reporter from the Louisville Courier Journal around Belmont. Enchanted as so many others had been, the reporter wrote:

> Its long, winding avenues, its playing fountains, its towers, rustic temples and statuary, numberless acacia arbors and retired sylvan seats, are to be found where a tete a tete can be enjoyed amid the perfume of the flowers, the shade of the trees and foliage and the cooling sounds of murmuring waters. In the lawn and garden are to be found rare and choice flowers from every country and every clime, and as their sweet exhilarating odors float through the atmosphere you wish that you could live in such a delightful place all your life.[35]

---

[33] Ibid., 23 December 1884
[34] Ibid., 27 July 1885.
[35] Louisville Courier-Journal, 18 May 1881, supplement.

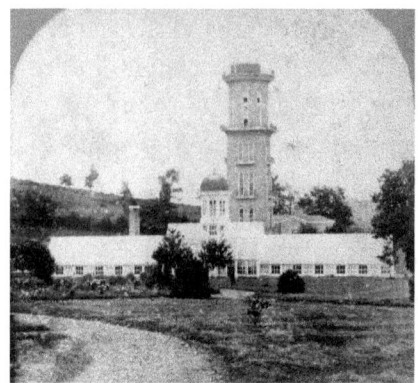 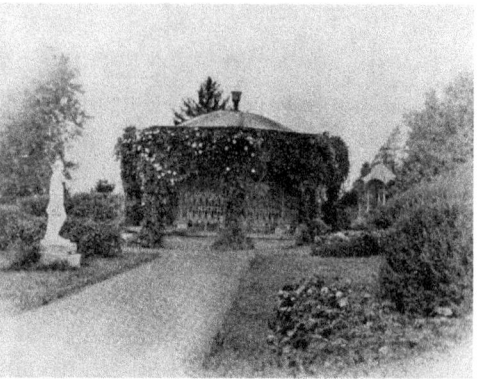

Left – Greenhouses, conservatory, and water tower.
Right – Center gazebo in the circular gardens.
Both images are from the collection of the Belmont Mansion Association.

Similar thoughts must have occurred to Cheatham, with his love of flowers, more than once; but it was not to last. In 1885 Adelicia moved with her daughter, Pauline, to Washington, D.C.[36] Her husband, who preferred to remain in Nashville and continue practicing medicine, moved into the Maxwell House Hotel in 1886.[37] On January 1, 1887, Adelicia sold Belmont mansion and its grounds of 78 acres to Lewis T. Baxter for $54,000. She also sold to Baxter all of her other Nashville property except her house on Cherry Street.[38]

In Washington, Adelicia, who was 70 years old on March 15, 1887, had begun building a house at 1776 Massachusetts Avenue. She and Pauline traveled to New York to buy furnishings for it in late April. The inclement weather caused Adelicia to become ill, and she died of pneumonia about ten days later on May 4, 1887. Dr. Jere Witherspoon preached her funeral held in Nashville's First Presbyterian Church. She was buried in Mt. Olivet Cemetery in a handsome Gothic mausoleum she had built in 1884 at a cost of $11,000, where her first two husbands and her deceased children were buried. Her obituary noted that she had been one of the most highly esteemed women in Nashville, occupying "a position that was hers by the possession of wealth, a strong intelligence, and a disposition of universal amiability."[39]

---

[36] Wardin, 31-32.
[37] Nashville City Directory, 1886.
[38] Wardin, 32.
[39] Ibid., The Daily American, 5 May 1867, 5.

In her last will and testament, dated January 22, 1884, Adelicia left the bulk of her estate to her sons William H. Acklen and Claude Acklen and to her daughter Pauline, noting that she did so by virtue of a marriage settlement which she had entered into with her husband, William A. Cheatham. She had already settled with her son Joseph H. Acklen in 1874, but also left him the 150-acre farm called Montvale, near her residence of Belle Monte, and a few personal effects. She left nothing to William A. Cheatham but did request that his son-in-law, Thomas S. Weaver, serve as Pauline's trustee. She appointed Anson Nelson executor of the will.

In a codicil dated January 22, 1887, after her move to Washington, Adelicia removed Thomas S. Weaver as trustee for Pauline and appointed in his stead her friend, James D. Porter, a former governor of Tennessee. In a second codicil dated April 29, 1887, in New York City, just days before her death on May 4th, Adelicia bequeathed to her daughter Pauline the house and furnishings in Washington, D.C., along with the funds to complete and furnish it "in the style and manner contemplated."[40]

Nothing was ever heard from the Cheatham family regarding the will. But Joseph H. Acklen contested it. He settled for $46,000 in cash or the equivalent and also received three promissory notes which he owed to his mother. Acklen further agreed to deliver to C. D. Berry, who was serving as administrator of the estate, a diamond ring valued at $3,000 and silver plate valued at $800, for which he would be reimbursed $3,800. In return, Joseph H. Acklen relinquished all other claims to the estate.[41]

Meanwhile, Adelicia's third husband was boarding at the Watkins Institute in 1887 while practicing medicine in partnership with his son, Richard. In 1888, he was boarding at Ichi-Nichi-Ni-San-Do, at 609 Church Street.[42] Thereafter he lived with his daughter and her husband, Mr. and Mrs. Thomas S. Weaver, who lived five miles out of Nashville on the Murfreesboro Pike, only a mile from the Tennessee Hospital for the Insane. He died at their home on June 9, 1900, at 11:30

---

[40] Davidson County Wills, vol. 30, pp. 155-164.
[41] Ibid.
[42] Nashville City Directory, 1888.

a.m., aged 80 years. His health had been remarkably good until the last few months of his life, when he sank into a gradual decline.

"Dr. Cheatham's death will cause genuine regret to his many friends, not only in Nashville, but throughout the state," one obituary read. "By his genial disposition and sincerity of manner he endeared himself to all. By inclination a student, he attained through application success and prominence in his profession. Not only in medicine, but in matters local and national, Dr. Cheatham was a student and unusually well posted on all current events."[43]

Unlike Adelicia, he did not leave a will, which probably indicates that he did not have an estate. But he had made a significant contribution to the life of his community as a physician and as a public servant. He died at an advanced age, having survived vicissitudes that might have destroyed a lesser man, "respected and admired for his professional ability and personal character,"[44] and described as "an aristocrat of the old school, a splendid type of the old-time gentleman."[45]

No doubt he would have appreciated those remarks. But if asked to appraise the crowning achievement of his professional career—to write his own obituary, in effect--he had, in a sense, done that prematurely in 1866 when he submitted his final report to the legislature of the State of Tennessee. In it he described how he had taken charge of

> the present center building standing alone on the back part of a bleak old field, on "Nubbin Ridge," with a belt of forest at one end, and the adjacent surface a succession of sinks and gullies. The lover of art or nature can scarcely [conceive] of a prospect more forbidding.   All the surroundings seemed so ordered as to invite, rather than to relieve, mental troubles and diseases. It was the nucleus of a benevolent institution of a great and liberal State, wherein I was born and reared; but means, taste, and energy were necessary for its development. I felt if the latter were made manifest the former would not be withheld; and the

---

[43] Nashville American, 11 June 1900, 8.
[44] Ibid.
[45] Ibid., 10 June 1900, 12.

result proved the correctness of my theory. I cultivated the taste necessary for my object by visiting, at my own expense, the oldest and most celebrated institutions in the United States, and expended my first year's salary thus, and in the purchase of material for the beginning of that system of ornamentation so extensively developed in after years. Public men began to perceive the benign influence of these decorations upon diseased mind, and what seemed at first, to many, as an inexcusable folly, the more observing soon appreciated as the highest wisdom. The blushing petals of a rare exotic would often rivet the attention of the incoherent mind, and restore normal reflection, while grosser objects would but excite scorn and disgust. The pivot upon which many a diseased mind has turned, and by slow degrees retrograded back to sanity, is revealed in as simple an object as a bird, a flower, or a picture.[46]

The Tennessee Hospital for the Insane had been his Belmont. He wrote lovingly of how the "old field" had gradually become

> a plain of green sward; and trees of green foliage, interspersed with rare and attractive flowers, were substituted for monotonous broom-sage; a morass was transformed into a lake; orchards were planted; extensive kitchen gardens and fields put in a high and remunerative state of cultivation. Greenhouses and fountains contributed their charming effects to the tout ensemble, and in sober propriety of language, a wilderness of broom-sage and briers, was made to blossom as a rose.

At the same time, he continued, new buildings were being erected in conformity with all the rules of hygiene, and incorporating the latest advances in heating, ventilation, and sewage, so that the Tennessee Hospital for the Insane "became, and was recognized at home and abroad, as among the first upon the continent."[47]

---

[46] Report of William A. Cheatham in <u>Appendix to Senate Journal</u>, 1865-66, 227-228.
[47] Ibid., 228.

He cited Sterling Cockrill, the dedicated president of the board, who had written, "The useful, the ornamental and elegant, are here blended in such nice proportions, as at once to excite the admiration and elevate our conceptions of human philanthropy."[48] Both statements are true. The project had been costly under Cheatham's administration; but the results had been universally applauded, and the State of Tennessee had earned from it a reputation for being enlightened, progressive, and humanitarian. In the post-war period, the State would no longer have the financial resources or the impetus to continue supporting the hospital on the scale established by Cheatham; and by the 1870s the era of optimism in psychiatry would yield to a less naive approach to mental illness, emphasizing the notion of incurability with less effort at providing therapy. For Tennesseans, Cheatham's administration as superintendent was a high water mark in state support of mental health until the administration of Frank Goad Clement as governor in the 1950s, a period of almost one hundred years.

Therefore, it is important that William A. Cheatham, M.D., not be remembered solely because he was the third and least visible of Adelicia Acklen's three husbands; he should not be defined in terms of her at all. They shared a love of beauty, both in nature as well as in art, and each built a magnificent estate. But she built hers for private use and entertainment, although she shared Belmont with a wide circle of friends and visitors; his was constructed no less lovingly for public philanthropy and out of humanitarian concern for the mentally ill.

---

[48] Ibid., 229.

BIBLIOGRAPHY

Books

American Psychiatric Association. <u>One Hundred Years of American Psychiatry</u>. New York: Columbia University Press, 1944.

Ash, Stephen v. <u>Middle Tennessee Society Transformed 1860-1870.</u> Baton Rouge: Louisiana State University Press, 1988.

<u>Biographical Directory, Tennessee General Assembly 1796-1967, Robertson County (Preliminary),</u> Tennessee State Library & Archives.

Brandau, Roberta Seawell, ed. <u>History of Homes and Gardens of Tennessee.</u> Nashville: Parthenon Press, 1936; reprint, Nashville: Friends of Cheekwood, 1964.

Brumbaugh, Thomas B., ed. <u>Architecture of Middle Tennessee: The Historic American Buildings Survey.</u> Nashville: Vanderbilt University Press, 1974.

Caplan, Ruth B. <u>Psychiatry and the Community in Nineteenth Century America.</u> New York: Basic Books, Inc., 1969.

Clayton, W. W. <u>History of Davidson County, Tennessee</u>. Philadelphia: 1880; reprint, Nashville: Charles Elder, 1971.

Connelly, Thomas Lawrence. <u>Army of the Heartland: The Army of Baton Rouge: Tennessee, 1861-62.</u> Louisiana State University Press, 1967.

Corlew, Robert E. <u>Tennessee, A Short History.</u> 2d ed. Knoxville: The University of Tennessee Press, 1984.

Craven, Avery O. <u>The Growth of Southern Nationalism, 1848-1861</u>. Vol. VI of <u>A History of the South</u>, Wendell Holmes Stephenson and E. Merton Coulter, eds. Baton Rouge: Louisiana State University Press, 1953.

Dain, Norman. <u>Concepts of Insanity in the United States, 1789-1865</u>. New Brunswick, NT: Rutgers University Press, 1964.

Deutsch, Albert. The Mentally Ill in America: A History of Their Care and Treatment from Colonial Times. 2d ed. New York: Columbia University Press, 1949.

Dokecki, Paul R., and Janice D, Mashburn. Beyond the Asylum: The History of Mental Handicap Policy in Tennessee, 1796-1948. Nashville: Tennessee Department of Mental Health and Retardation, 1984.

Duke, Basil Wilson. History of Morgan's Cavalry. Cincinnati: Miami Printing, 1867; reprint, Bloomington: Indiana University Press, 1960.

Durham, Walter T. Nashville: The Occupied City (The First Seventeen Months--February 16, 1862, to June 30, 1863). Nashville: Tennessee Historical Society, 1985.

_____. Reluctant Partners: Nashville and the Union, July 1, 1863, to June 30, 1865. Nashville: Tennessee Historical Society, 1987.

Eaton, Clement. A History of the Old South. New York: The Macmillan Company, 1949.

Fitch, John. Annals of the Cumberland. Philadelphia: J.B. Lippincott & Company, 1864.

Goodspeed Histories of Montgomery, Robertson, Humphreys, Stewart, Dickson, Cheatham, Houston Counties of Tennessee. Columbia, Tennessee: 1975.

Graf, LeRoy P., and Ralph w. Haskins, eds. The Papers of Andrew Johnson. 6 vols. to date. Knoxville: University of Tennessee Press, 1967-.

Grob, Gerald N. Edward Jarvis and the Medical World of Nineteenth Century America. Knoxville: University of Tennessee Press, 1978.

_____. Mental Institutions in America, Social Policy to 1875. New York: The Free Press, 1973.

_____. The State Hospital and the Mentally Ill: A History of Worchester State Hospital in Massachusetts. Chapel Hill: University of North Carolina Press, 1966.

Hall, Clifton R. <u>Andrew Johnson, Military Governor of Tennessee.</u> Princeton: 1916.

Henderson, Deborah Kelley. <u>Robertson County's Heritage of Homes</u>. Springfield: Robertson County Antiquities Foundation, 1979.

Holland, Cecil Fletcher. <u>Morgan and His Raiders: A Biography of the Confederate General</u>. New York: Macmillan, 1942.

Horn, Stanley F. <u>Tennessee's War, 1861-1865.</u> Nashville: Tennessee Civil War Centennial Commission, 1965.

Hughes, Mary B. <u>Hearthstones: The Story of Historic Rutherford County Homes.</u> Murfreesboro: Mid-South Publishing co., 1942.

<u>Index to Interments in the Nashville City Cemetery.</u> Nashville: Tennessee State Library and Archives, 1964.

Kennedy, Roger J. <u>Architecture, Men, Women and Money in America 1600- 1860</u>. New York: Random House, 1985.

Love, Charles H. <u>Springfield's First 100 Years</u>, Robertson County Times, n.d.

Marshall, Helen E. <u>Dorothea Dix, Forgotten Samaritan</u>. Chapel Hill: University of North Carolina Press, 1937.

McGovern, Constance M. <u>Masters of Madness: Social Origins of the American Psychiatric Profession</u>. Hanover, NH: University Press of New England, 1985.

<u>Nashville City Directory</u>, 1867-1890.

Norwood, William Frederick. <u>Medical Education in the United States Before the Civil War</u>. New York: Arno Press and the New York Times, 1971.

<u>Obsequies of John L, Cheatham, M.D. of Nashville, Tennessee, with an address by J. B, Ferguson</u>. Nashville: John T, s. Fall, 1863.

Patton, James Welch. Unionism and Reconstruction in Tennessee, 1860-1868. 2d ed. Chapel Hill: University of North Carolina Press, 1934.

Ramage, James A. Rebel Raider: The Life of General John Hunt Morgan. Lexington: University Press of Kentucky, 1986.

Randall, James G., and David Donald. The Civil War and Reconstruction. Boston: Heath, 1961.

Rosenberg, Charles E. The Trial of the Assassin Guiteau: Psychiatry and Law in the Gilded Age. Chicago: University of Chicago Press, 1968.

Rothman, David J. The Discovery of the Asylum: Social Order and Disorder in the New Republic. Boston: Little, Brown and Company, 1971.

Simon, John Y., ed. The Personal Memoirs of Julia Dent Grant (Mrs. Ulysses s. Grant). New York: G. P, Putnam's Sons, 1975.

Stephenson, Wendell Holmes. Isaac Franklin, Slave Trader and Planter of the Old South. Baton Rouge: Louisiana State University Press, 1938; reprint, Gloucester, Massachusetts: Peter Smith, 1968.

Swiggert, Howard. The Rebel Raider: A Life of John Hunt Morgan. Indianapolis: Bobbs-Merrill, 1934.

Thomas, Miss Jane H. Old Days in Nashville, Tenn.: Reminiscences. Reprinted from the Nashville Daily American, 1895, 96. Nashville, Tenn.: Publishing House Methodist Episcopal Church, South, 1897.

Wardin, Albert W., Jr. Belmont Mansion, The Home of Joseph and Adelicia Acklen. Nashville: Historic Belmont Association, 1981.

Wilson, Dorothy Clarke. Stranger and Traveler: The Story of Dorothea Dix, American Reformer. Boston: Little, Brown and Company, 1975.

Woodward, C. Vann. Thinking Back: The Perils of Writing History. Baton Rouge: Louisiana State University Press, 1986.

ARTICLES

"American Hospitals for the Insane." North American Review 79 (July 1854): 66-90.

Ash, Stephen V. "Sharks in an Angry Sea: Civilian Resistance and Guerilla Warfare in Occupied Middle Tennessee, 1862-1865." Tennessee Historical Quarterly XLV, No. 3 (Fall 1986): 217-229.

Bockoven, J. Sanbourne. "Moral Treatment in American Psychiatry." Journal of Nervous and Mental Disease 124 No. 2 (August 1956): 167-194; No. 3 (September 1956): 292-309.

Davis, Louise. "Belmont Mystery Unravels." The Tennessean Magazine, October 1978, 20-24.

Graham, Eleanor. "Belmont: 1. Nashville Home of Adelicia Acklen." Tennessee Historical Quarterly Vol. XXX, No. 4 (Winter 1971): 345-368.

Horn, Stanley F. "Nashville During the Civil War." Tennessee Historical Quarterly 4 (1945): 3-22.

Kiser, John. "Scion of Belmont." Tennessee Historical Quarterly Vol. XXXVIII, No. 1 (Spring 1979): 34-61.

"Scion of Belmont, Part II." Tennessee Historical Quarterly Vol. XXXVIII, No. 2, (Summer 1979): 188- 203.

Luton, Frank, M.D., and Charles E. Goshen, M.D. "A Brief History of Tennessee Psychiatry." Journal of the Tennessee Medical Association 65 (8) (August 1972): 708-715.

Maslowski, Peter. "From Reconciliation to Reconstruction :Lincoln, Johnson, and Tennessee." Tennessee Historical Quarterly XLII (1983): 281-98; 343-61.

Spain, Rufus B. "R, B. C Howell: Nashville Baptist Leader in the Civil War Period." Tennessee Historical Quarterly XIV (1955): 323-340.

Thompson, E. Bruce. "Reforms in the Care of the Insane in Tennessee, 1830-1850." Tennessee Historical Quarterly III (4) (December 1944): 319-334.

Warr, Otis S. "The History of Medical Education in Tennessee." The Centennial History of the Tennessee State Medical Association 1830-1930. Philip M, Hamer, ed. Nashville: Tennessee State Medical Association, 1930.

JOURNALS

American Journal of Insanity IX-XX (1852-1864).

Bowling, w. K., M.D., and Paul F, Eve, M.D., eds. The Nashville Journal of Medicine and Surgery 1-21 (February 1851-1861).

House Journal of the First Session of the 33rd General Assembly of the State of Tennessee, Convened at Nashville October 1859. Nashville: E.G. Eastman & co., 1859.

Proceedings of the Medical Society of the State of Tennessee at the 16th Annual Meeting. Nashville: Cameron & Fall, 1845.

Proceedings of the Medical Society of the State of Tennessee at the 17th Annual Meeting. Nashville: Burton, Billings & Fall, 1846.

Proceedings of the Medical Convention of the State of Tennessee. Nashville: E. R. Glascock & Co., 1847.

Proceedings of the 21st Annual Meeting of the Tennessee Medical Society. Murfreesboro: April, 1850.

Transactions of the Tennessee Medical Society. Nashville: J. F. Morgan, 1853.

Transactions of the 27th Annual Session of the Tennessee Medical Society. Nashville: Cameron & Fall, 1856.

Transactions of the 29th Annual Meeting of the Tennessee Medical Society. Nashville: T. s. Fall, 1858.

REPORTS

Reports of the Trustees, Treasurer and Physician of the Tennessee Hospital for the Insane, Transmitted to the Legislature on the Sixth November, 1853. Nashville: Union and American Steam Press, 1853.

Second Biennial Reports of the Trustees, Treasurer, and the Physician and Superintendent of the Tennessee Hospital for the Insane. Nashville: B. R. McKennie & Co., 1855,

Third Biennial Reports of the Trustees, Treasurer, Architect, and the Physician and Superintendent of the Tennessee Hospital for the Insane. Nashville: G. C. Torbett & Co., 1857.

Fourth Biennial Reports of the Trustees, Treasurer, and the Superintendent and Physician of the Tennessee Hospital for the Insane. Nashville: E. G. Eastman & Co., 1859.

Reports of the Trustees and Superintendent of the Tennessee Hospital for the Insane, presented to the General Assembly April 3, 1865. Nashville: John T. S. Fall, 1865.

Tennessee. Appendix to the Senate Journal. 1865-66.

RECORDS

Acklen, Adelicia, and William A. Cheatham. Marriage contract, 17 June 1867. Davidson County, Tennessee, Deed Book 38: 287-9.

Acklen, Adelicia. 155-164, 489. Will. Davidson County, Tennessee, Wills, Vol. 30: Final settlement: see Minute Book Y: 283.

Davidson County, Tennessee, Chancery Court Minute Book Q: 468-470.

_____. Chancery court Minute Book U: 52-53, 360-362.

_____. Chancery Court Minute Book V: 90-91.

"Records of the U.S. Army Commands." Record Group 393. National Archives. Washington, D,C.

"Union Provost Marshals File of Papers Relating to Individual Civilians." Record Group 109. National Archives. Washington, D.C.

U.S. War Department. The War of the Rebellion: A Compilation of the Official Records of the Union and Confederate Armies. Series II, Vol. V. Washington, D.C.: Government Printing Office, 1899.

NEWSPAPERS

Dorsey, A. L. "Historical Events of Past Hundred Years." Undated clipping from the collection of James Henry Taylor, Springfield, Tennessee.

Louisville Courier-Journal, 18 May 1881 (supplement).

Nashville American, 10, 11 June 1900: 8, 12; 15 August 1909 (Magazine Section): 3; 22 August 1909.

Nashville Daily American, 5 May 1867: 5; 31 August 1877: 4; 5 May 1887: 5; 8 May 1887: 7; 31 May 1888: 6; 15 March 1889: 5.

Nashville Republican Banner, 16 December 1866: 3; 19 December 1866: 4.

Nashville Union and American, 22 May 1872: 4.

Nashville Weekly American, 11 May 1887: 3.

Newspaper clipping, 1867, in scrapbook owned by Dr. Mack Wayne Craig, Nashville.

UNPUBLISHED MATERIALS

Ackland, William Hayes. Autobiography. Southern Historical Collection, University of North Carolina, Chapel Hill.

Brown, Mark, Virginia Graves, John Lancaster. *Adelicia Acklen's Life in Chronological Order*. Unpublished manuscript in Belmont Mansion research files. 2018

Cheatham-Ready family papers in the possession of Mrs. H. Clinton Parrent and Mrs. Charles Bradley, Nashville.

Correspondence of Adelicia Acklen Cheatham, McGavock Hayes Papers, Tennessee State Library & Archives.

Correspondence of Adelicia Acklen Cheatham and William B. Lawrence Diary, Lawrence Family Papers, Tennessee State Library & Archives.

Crabb, Alfred Leland. "The Acts of Adelicia." Old Oak Club Papers, Tennessee State Library & Archives.

Hardison, Edwin T, "In the Toils of War: Andrew Johnson and the Federal Occupation of Tennessee." Ph.D. dissertation, University of Tennessee at Knoxville, 1981.

Letter of Emma Y. Player, 24 June 1866, Yeatman-Polk Papers, Tennessee State Library & Archives.

Letters of Annie L. Pope, 19 December 1866; Sarah Rachel Polk Jones, 18 February 1867; Emily Donelson Polk Williams, 25 February 1867; and Mary Brown Polk Yeatman, c. 1867, in Brown, Campbell, and Richard Stoddert Ewell Papers, Tennessee State Library & Archives.

Letters of William A. Cheatham to Dorothea L. Dix, 18 December 1851; 14 January, 10 February, 2 December, 1859. Houghton Library of Harvard University.

Morgan, John Hunt. Papers. Department of Special Collections, Manuscripts, Western Kentucky University, Bowling Green.

_____. Papers. Southern Historical Collection, University of North Carolina, Chapel Hill.

Ramage, James A., to Kay Baker Gaston, 16 May 1988, in possession of author.

Ready, C. Alice. Diary. Southern Historical Collection, University of North Carolina, Chapel Hill.

Ready family papers in the possession of Andrew c. Buddenhagen, Murfreesboro.

Washington family papers, Tennessee State Library and Archives, Nashville.

INTERVIEWS

Chester, Bettie Thomas. Interviews by author. 1988-1989.

Parrent, Mary W., and Martha W. Bradley. Interview by author, 27 April 1988.

Proctor, Mrs. David Y. Interview by author.

Wills, Irene Jackson. Interview by author (telephone), 6 April 1988.

REFERENCE

Malone, Dumas, ed. *Dictionary of American Biography*. Vols. XIII, XX. New York: Charles Scribner's Sons, 1934.

www.ingramcontent.com/pod-product-compliance
Lightning Source LLC
Chambersburg PA
CBHW051454290426
44109CB00016B/1752